David Reavely

the BIG FAT MYSTERY

MILLIONS OF PEOPLE'S
ATTEMPTS TO LOSE WEIGHT
ARE THWARTED BY HIDDEN
FOOD INTOLERANCES. UNCOVER
YOURS AND GET THE
HEALTHY BODY YOU WANT.

Published by Metro, an imprint of John Blake Publishing Ltd,
3 Bramber Court, 2 Bramber Road,
London W14 9PB, England

www.blake.co.uk

First published in paperback in 2008

ISBN 978 1 84454 575 9

British Library Cataloguing-in-Publication Data:

A catalogue record for this book is available from the British Library.

Design by www.envydesign.co.uk

Printed and bound in Great Britain by CPI Bookmarque, Croydon CR0 4TD

1 3 5 7 9 10 8 6 4 2

Papers used by John Blake Publishing are natural, recyclable products made from wood
grown in sustainable forests. The manufacturing processes conform to the environmental
regulations of the country of origin.

Every attempt has been made to contact the relevant copyright-holders, but some were
unobtainable. We would be grateful if the appropriate people could contact us.

This publication is designed to provide health educational data in regard to the subject
covered. It is a reference and experiential work of general interest and benefit to readers and is
not intended to treat, diagnose or prescribe. The information contained herein is in no way to
be considered a substitute for consultation with a competent health care professional. If
pregnant or breastfeeding, you should consult a qualified doctor or health practitioner before
embarking on the application of nutritional advice in this book. Skilled medical opinion is
advised on specific health complaints before any course of action is taken.

I would like to dedicate this book to the memory of my parents, who always encouraged and supported me in my learning endeavours. Also, to my sister Iris, brother-in-law Jackie and my nieces, Michelle and Yvonnne, who, along with my son, Adam, and daughter, Josie, have shared in my nutritional voyage of discovery.

Foreword

In this fantastic book, Dave Reavely has again shown tremendous knowledge of one of the most significant problems we are faced with in Great Britain today, the growing prevalence of overweight and obesity. He has studied this subject as a sportsman for many years, has written several books on good dietary management, and this practical and life-enhancing guide will equip you to enjoy a healthier life.

In Dave's easy to follow programme he offers plenty of advice on how to think positively and tackle the problem. I am sure this book will be a success for many people who struggle with their weight.

Jan de Vries, former health guru on Richard and Judy's *This Morning* and *Open House with Gloria Hunniford*

Contents

Part II

Acknowledgements

Many thanks to all my friends, family and colleagues, who through their tireless support encouraged me to write this book.

I am also indebted to Raymond Francis MSC, Dr Douglas N Graham and YorkTest Laboratories, who gave their permission to use extracts from their work.

Thanks also to world-renowned naturopath and author, Jan de Vries, who has been a huge source of support and encouragement over many years.

Finally, I am so grateful to my partner, Jenny, who gave me much-needed technical support and was a true source of inspiration.

Introduction

The chances are that you picked up this book because you have a problem with regulating your weight. Maybe you've been on that yo-yo diet bandwagon when you initially lose a few extra pounds only to regain whatever you've lost as soon as you return to your usual eating patterns. Perhaps you've reached the stage, possibly not for the first time, where you've hit the proverbial 'brick wall' when no matter how much you exercise and do all of the things that are supposed to be effective, nothing budges. If you happen to be one of those 'tried everything' people, then take heart because this book might just provide you with the solution you've been looking for: namely, that hidden food intolerances could be blocking your attempts to shed those excess pounds!

As a nutritional therapist who specialises in food intolerance testing, I've encountered numerous overweight men and women who had already accepted defeat in the battle of the bulge. In fact, many of them were being tested for intolerances because they had other health issues such as an irritable bowel, bloated stomach, frequent headaches or a skin condition that refused to respond to treatment. A large percentage tested positive for one or more foods. Once they began to exclude the offending food (or foods) from their diet, their symptoms often cleared up. This in itself was a brilliant achievement – however, it wasn't the only thing to happen. Much to their surprise (and mine too in the early days), they began to lose excess weight. Not only did they lose weight, they were also shedding pounds without having to count calories. Pretty soon the truth of the matter began to emerge: somehow being intolerant to one or more foods could result in an inability to lose excess weight! At the time I didn't understand the nature of the biological mechanisms behind this amazing phenomenon, all I knew was that when a person with a food intolerance eliminated the food to which they had become over-sensitive, they would often lose weight and frequently after years of unsuccessful dieting. What's more, provided they ate sensibly and continued to avoid the offending food, the weight would stay off, unlike in the past.

At this stage, the inevitable question was this: how many people with weight regulation problems also have hidden food intolerance? The answer, as I discovered, is a lot more than is commonly realised. When writing this book it was always my intention to highlight how food intolerances can interfere with the body's attempts to lose excess weight. Nevertheless, it's important to be aware that there is a bigger picture and that food intolerances are merely an outward symptom of a deeper systemic condition which, when addressed, can result in an overall improvement in health, a lowered propensity to develop intolerances and a heightened ability to effectively regulate weight. That's why this book focuses on the whole person and not just the issue of food intolerance since one can impact on the other.

In Part I, I explain how I became aware of the direct connection between food intolerances and weight gain. I have also provided an explanation of the difference between food intolerance and food allergy before focusing my attention on four major food intolerances: wheat, gluten, dairy and yeast (the latter sometimes being an indication of a yeast overgrowth known as *candidiasis*). At the end of each chapter on the major intolerances, you will find a comprehensive list of recipes designed to provide a choice of healthy, balanced meals for the food intolerance sufferer. There is also a chapter on the less headline-grabbing food intolerances before we deal with the subject of food rotation. The final chapter in this part of the book helps you choose the right tests to identify your food intolerances.

In Part II, I offer an explanation of what causes food intolerance before addressing what factors predispose us towards its development in the first place. Here, I have focused attention on what I perceive to be the major influences: among them a high level of toxicity within the body, the importance of a healthy diet, the role of healthy fats in relation to weight loss, how to strengthen the immune system and the importance of healing the gut and reducing inflammation. Finally, we conclude with an action plan which takes into account all these factors and represents a nutritional and lifestyle prescription designed to alleviate – and in some cases reverse – food intolerances, reduce inflammation, promote good health and permanent weight loss.

For those of you who decide to give my action plan a go, remember that it is important to be consistent. Don't expect overnight results. If you persevere with the plan, however, and initiate the necessary lifestyle changes, you have every chance of being rewarded with an increased ability to regulate your weight, and the added bonus of improved all-round health.

Dave Reavely Cert Ed. Bed (Hon), DN Med, MBANT

All eggs are large, organic
All butter is unsalted
All herbs fresh, unless otherwise stated
All chocolate is dark (min 70% cocoa solids), unless stated
All measurements are approximate, with cup measurements
rounded to the nearest quarter where appropriate

Part I

1

Food intolerances and weight problems: the story unfolds

I guess you could say that my initiation into the world of food allergies and intolerances started early in life. When I was in my teens I made the discovery that I was reacting to a whole host of everyday foods. How did I know? Well, just cause and effect really! Whenever I ate a slice of bread, my joints would become painful and inflamed but when I stopped eating bread, lo and behold, the symptoms disappeared. Mind you, this turned out to be slightly more complicated than simply eliminating the proverbial 'staff of life' from my diet. Think in terms of all grains (yes, even rice), potatoes, pulses, nuts, meat and fish, and you begin to get the picture. Eating any one of those foods was enough to transform me from an athletic sports-loving teenager into the equivalent of a hobbling geriatric in one fell swoop. So, you can imagine what a combination of those foods would do.

OK, you may well ask, so what was left for you to eat? Well, let's just say that it was lucky that I liked fruits and vegetables because most of my diet revolved around their consumption on a daily basis. Also, I was able to consume some dairy products in the form of goat's milk and yoghurts. This provided me with enough protein, and being so much into my sports I really needed it. Of course on the plus side, eating such large volumes of these foods kept me fit and healthy. In fact, as long as I didn't stray from my diet, I was mostly pain-free. To this day my diet is still based around fruits and vegetables, and now, in the light of current knowledge on the protein content of fruits and vegetables, I realise that I get enough protein purely from these sources.

Not surprisingly, years later when I began work as a nutritional advisor for a company that carried out food intolerance tests, my early experiential grounding in food intolerances was to prove invaluable. There I was, dealing with people who were testing positive for wheat, gluten and dairy intolerance, with a number of clients who had yeast infections thrown in for good measure! During that time I worked with the owner of the business, who also happened to do the testing. My job was to interpret the test results that appeared on a computer screen and then create a dietary programme for the client.

An amazing discovery!
The more experience I gained from observing the results of dozens of health-screening tests, the more I began to enjoy my work. I soon realised that helping people make a big difference to their health was a hugely rewarding business. The fact was that those previously suffering from a diverse range of symptoms were gradually able to regain control of their health and ultimately, their lives. Without wishing to sound too sensationalist, provided clients adhered to the diet programme, I have witnessed some pretty astounding

improvements over the years. These include the complete disappearance of eczema, migraines, depression (including manic depression), Irritable Bowel Syndrome (IBS) and other digestive problems, elimination of arthritic pain, improved concentration, elimination of sinus problems, disappearance of menstrual difficulties and reduced hyperactivity in children. Generally speaking, most people reported a big improvement in their energy levels too!

All of this was impressive in itself, but in addition to these significant improvements, I began to notice that something else was happening. A lot of clients who were overweight reported back that just a few days into the programme they were losing weight and some would lose as much as half a stone in the first week. This initial weight loss gradually slowed down as the weeks progressed but nevertheless, it would often continue for a while. However, one thing was for sure: not only were these people feeling in much better health, with less colds, fewer aches and pains and more energy, it was almost as if someone had flicked the 'ON' switch for their metabolism. Suddenly they were digesting food more easily and regulating their weight was much simpler. Remember, some of them had struggled with weight problems for years. So, I began to ask myself the question: what was happening? As you'll discover in Chapter 2, the answer may have implications for those thousands of people who suffer from obesity.

2

How food intolerances can block your attempts to lose weight

What really astounded me about some clients was their rapid and significant weight loss over the first couple of weeks into the dietary programme. A typical case might be someone who tests positive for gluten intolerance. Let's call this imaginary client John. This was how the story would often unfold...

How water retention got my attention
Having started his gluten-free diet, John noticed that the bloating and indigestion he used to suffer was beginning to disappear. Obviously he was delighted about this, but it wasn't unexpected because I had already explained to him that an improvement in his condition was likely. What was surprising, however, was the fact that he reported a significant loss in weight. In fact, just over two weeks into the diet he had lost around ten pounds! This was despite the fact that in the past he'd tried every weight-loss diet imaginable and nothing had worked. On this occasion, the only thing he'd done differently was to eliminate gluten from

his diet. He was delighted with this rather unexpected turn of events.

Naturally, he was curious as to how the elimination of one type of food from his diet should have such a dramatic effect on his weight. One clue emerged from an improvement in another of his health conditions: apart from his original digestive problems, John also suffered from oedema (water retention). Often his ankles would swell up at the end of the day and his legs felt heavy and tender to touch. Just one week into the gluten-free diet he noticed that his ankles were no longer swollen. Seemingly, he was losing excess fluid. This was my first real clue that the initial weight loss experienced by clients like John was due to a loss of fluid from the body. Later I was to discover that the presence of a food intolerance resulted in the body retaining fluid to dilute the effects of the offending substance that it identifies as a toxin.

Although in this case John is a fictitious character, when it comes to helping clients with their weight problems the foregoing scenario typifies the kind of situation that I encounter on a regular basis. Sometimes these are people who I encounter on a casual basis, such as a retired gentleman who trains in my local gym. (See Barry's story, opposite)

Why calories are not the Arch Enemy

The aforementioned patient serves to illustrate that once intolerant foods are identified and removed from the diet then the caloric consumption is not necessarily the key factor influencing weight loss. This is because the initial loss of fluid is followed by an improvement in the body's metabolism. Perhaps for the first time in years the patient may discover that they are digesting foods much more efficiently. This not only involves a more thorough breakdown of protein,

Barry's story

Despite the fact that he'd tried every remedy going, Barry had a big problem with blocked sinuses that he had been unable to resolve. I asked him to keep a food diary and deduced from this that he was likely to be suffering from dairy and wheat intolerance. When he omitted them from his diet his sinuses gradually cleared for the first time in many years. However, being around twenty-one pounds overweight, he was delighted when his new way of eating resulted in the loss of fourteen pounds in the first six weeks. I wasn't in the least bit surprised, having witnessed this kind of result many times over the years. In fact, I believe there are many thousands of obese people who would experience similar results if only they could identify and eradicate their food intolerances.

Michael Rosenbaum, M.D., who runs an allergy clinic in Mill Valley, California, has observed similar results in terms of initial water loss followed by fat loss. He states: 'Food sensitivities can cause the body to retain both water and fat.' When it comes to the subject of calories, Rosenbaum cites the example of one of his patients who seemed to defy the concept of reducing caloric consumption to sustain weight. This gentleman was found to be sensitive to dairy products and decided to substitute bread and beer to make up for the removal of milk and cheese from his diet. It's likely that he was probably consuming even more calories but still managed to lose ten pounds in the first month without even trying. The next time Rosenbaum saw him, his trousers were practically falling off!

carbohydrates and fats but also an improved ability in the digestive system to absorb nutrients from food. It's a little like releasing the floodgates in a dam. Suddenly, after years of unsuccessful dieting and endless hours of exercise, the weight begins to diminish.

How food addiction can result in weight gain

Have you ever experienced cravings for a certain food? For example, many people crave bread. If you suggest they might have wheat or gluten intolerance, they go into defensive mode! They refuse to contemplate life without bread and other wheat-based products. Could it be that they have an addiction to the foods they are sensitive to? The answer is: absolutely yes! This is because eating the food you are sensitive to makes you feel temporarily better. When that food is withdrawn, you begin to feel uncomfortable. So, like a drug addict who needs his next fix, you eat more of the same food to alleviate the 'withdrawal' symptoms. As Stephen Levine, Ph.D, writes in his excellent article 'Food Addiction, Food Allergy and Overweight', 'Obese people can testify to the overwhelming power of food allergy addiction. Compulsive eaters crave and continue to eat those allergenic foods to which they are addicted day after day.' Frequently, the obese person does not realise that daily food cravings or eating habits are based on a physiological need to halt withdrawal symptoms caused by food allergy addiction.

The good news is that when food sensitivity is identified and the offending food is eradicated from the diet, cravings gradually diminish and often disappear altogether.

How food addiction can affect the brain

Have you ever wondered why some people with food allergies

and intolerances end up binge eating? In some cases sufferers describe these foods as leaving them feeling quite tired or even dopey. Others may describe a feeling of euphoria. In this way the food acts as a psychological 'safety valve'. In other words, it can relieve the pressure we feel when experiencing uncomfortable situations. We sometimes refer to this type of situation as 'comfort eating'.

But what is the mechanism behind this process? To understand what happens we need to know a little about endorphins. Endorphins are the feel-good chemicals produced by the brain. Not only do they make us feel good, but they also act as natural painkillers. They do this by binding onto receptor sites that cause us pain and switching on pleasant feelings. Drugs such as opiates (e.g. morphine) also bind onto these receptor sites, which is why they are effective painkillers. Some scientists believe that endorphin-like substances are produced from the digestion of foods such as wheat, milk and corn. Are you starting to get the picture? That's right, these endorphin-like substances have been shown to latch onto the endorphin receptor sites resulting in short-term positive feelings. Of course when the effect wears off, we end up craving our endorphin 'fix'. Hence the binge-eating merry-go-round continues and with it an increasing problem with obesity. In addition to the endorphin effect it is also known that wheat contains opiate-like substances and that is another possible reason why it can become such an addictive food.

CAUTION!

In my experience many of the people who begin to eliminate an offending food (or foods) from their diet fall into two categories. Let's call these categories A and B. The person who belongs in category A often begins to experience an improvement in their condition as soon as they omit the foods they are intolerant to and this may happen after only a day or two. In comparison, the person who belongs to category B may feel worse initially, followed by a steady improvement thereafter. Clients often ask me why this is the case. I have concluded that in the case of the category B type person, the body seizes the opportunity to detoxify itself. Hence the reason why they may feel a little worse at first, followed by an improvement in their health – a pattern commonly observed when someone implements positive changes in their eating habits.

A good example would be a person who suffers from mucous congestion. He/she may experience an increased discharge of mucous, perhaps in the form of a succession of head colds. This happened to a friend of mine who for many years suffered from sinus problems. However, having omitted dairy produce and gluten from his diet, he was pain-free for the first time in as long as he could remember. Also, not only did he lose a considerable amount of weight, his sense of smell also returned. However, at first his body, no longer burdened by the allergens, began to purge itself of all the mucous that had caused him so much pain and misery over the years.

THE BIG **FAT** MYSTERY

So how can we break free of this reliance on the very food (or foods) that we are reacting to and therefore regain control of our body's ability to regulate weight properly? The following steps will help you get back on track:

- Have yourself tested to identify if you are sensitive to any foods in your diet.
- Omit the offending food (or foods) from your diet for one month. This should give you time to evaluate how you are responding.
- Aim to exercise on a regular basis since this encourages the brain to release endorphins, which should help you to break free from the foods you are addicted to.

Withdrawal symptoms

Irrespective of whether you fall into category A or B, suffering from uncomfortable symptoms can sometimes be the result of withdrawal symptoms. When the offending foods are removed from your diet, it's just like removing a drug to which you are addicted and you may experience a worsening of your original symptoms. It usually takes about five days before you come through this.

Summary

When a person removes foods they are intolerant to from their diet, the following positive effects often take place:

- Metabolism and digestive system normalise
- Brain chemistry normalises
- Food addictions and cravings disappear
- Water retention disappears.

3

Allergies and intolerances: what's the difference?

Not surprisingly, many people get confused over the difference between allergies and intolerances. Basically, an allergy occurs when the body becomes over-sensitive to a food or other substance. For instance, when we eat a food that we are sensitive to, the body over-reacts to its presence in the body. In simple terms, it's an exaggerated and misguided defensive reaction by the body's immune system to something that is normally harmless. When this happens the immune system produces 'markers' (antibodies) identifying the substances that the body doesn't like. There are several different types of antibody, namely, IgE, IgG, IgA, IgM and IgD. The primary antibody relating to so-called classic allergies is the IgE antibody. When someone with a classic food allergy ingests the food they are sensitive to, the immune system responds in the following manner:

- First, the offending food (known as allergen) is eaten (e.g. wheat)
- The immune system is alerted to make IgE antibodies

specific to that food. Millions of these IgE antibodies circulate in the blood and combine with the specific food

- The resulting IgE molecule then combines with mast cells which are embedded in the body's solid tissues at sites such as the lining of the lungs, nasal passages and the walls of the intestines
- The IgE molecule triggers the mast cell to release histamine and other chemicals that result in classic allergy symptoms such as gastrointestinal upsets, swollen throat, sinusitis, etc.

If the allergen enters the body through the lungs (e.g. pollen) or is absorbed through the skin (e.g. printer's ink), then this may result in allergic reactions such as skin rashes, asthma, hay fever, etc. All of these reactions are immediate inflammatory reactions and are referred to as Type 1 allergic reactions. In essence, those who experience allergic reactions are often well aware of what upsets them and therefore find it easy to identify the source of the problem.

Food intolerances

Some reactions to food do not involve IgE antibodies. They are sometimes referred to as 'intolerances' or 'sensitivities'. In contrast to the quick reactions associated with allergies, the effects of an intolerance may manifest themselves a few hours later or in some cases even a day or two later. That being the case, you can imagine how intolerances are much more difficult to discern than allergies. In fact if you have several intolerances it can be a bit of a nightmare to try and sort out which food is affecting you and which isn't! Some are the result of the body's inability to digest the food in question – for instance, some people find it difficult to digest lactose (milk sugar) in milk. This is usually because they lack the lactose-digesting enzyme, lactase. In such a situation, if the lactase-deficient person consumes milk, they experience uncomfortable digestive symptoms such as bloating and indigestion. However, leaving this type of food intolerance aside, it is now thought that some delayed intolerances are associated with another kind of marker known as IgG antibodies. These antibodies also attach themselves to allergens, but only result in symptoms when they reach a certain level in the body.

Experience has taught me that there are many people who suffer from environmental and food intolerances, including babies and infants. Two of the most common problems that I encounter on a daily basis are dairy and grain intolerances. Wheat intolerance is quite common, as is intolerance to gluten, which is the protein component in wheat, barley, rye and oats. Gluten is composed of a combination of two proteins, glutelin and gliadin. Numerous studies have identified gliadin as the intestinal irritant. However, oats don't contain it, which is why some gluten-sensitive people can tolerate them. Those who can't may be reacting to other proteins present in oats or possibly to cross-contamination with gluten milled in the same grain-processing factory.

The more clients tested positive for food intolerances over the years, the more I realised the diverse range of health problems that they can cause. I used to think food intolerances mainly affected the digestive system resulting in symptoms such as bloating, indigestion, acid reflux, constipation and Irritable Bowel Syndrome. Boy, was I in for a big surprise! It wasn't very long before I realised that these conditions were just the tip of the iceberg. For a start, some clients didn't experience any digestive problems at all. Or if they did, they were also suffering from some other complaint such as migraines, depression or a skin condition which they didn't connect with their digestive problems. In essence, the range of conditions often included the following:

- Eczema
- Psoriasis
- Migraines
- Attention Deficit Disorder (ADD)
- Poor memory
- Depression
- Low energy
- Bedwetting
- Hay fever
- Arthritis

- Muscle aches
- Menstrual problems
- Sinus congestion
- Rhinitis
- Behavioural problems and hyperactivity in children
- Mood swings
- Erratic sleep patterns
- Mouth ulcers
- Weight gain

The list is far from exhaustive and does not include digestive problems that are sometimes, but not always, present. What astounded me was the fact that quite a few of these people were being treated for their conditions with drugs, usually without any long-term success. This was not surprising considering that the underlying cause was not being identified: i.e. intolerance to food, or more than one food. Remember, this also included people who had been struggling to control their weight problems, sometimes over several years.

> ## IMPORTANT
>
> If you suffer from any of these health conditions, then it might be worth being tested for food intolerances. For details of organisations that conduct testing, see the Useful Information section at the end of this book. Support for those adhering to an exclusion diet is available on my website www.fooddetective.co.uk.

Frequently asked questions about food intolerances

Over the years I have been asked many questions about food intolerances. I have included some of the most frequently asked questions below:

Question: What is gluten?
Answer: It is a type of protein present in wheat, barley, rye and oats. This protein is made from two components: glutelin and gliadin. It is the gliadin component that people can become sensitive to. Having said this, the gliadin component is absent from oats, which is why some gluten-sensitive people can tolerate them.

Question: Why do so many people suffer from wheat and gluten intolerances these days?
Answer: I believe this is due to the amount of wheat (which is also highest in gluten) that most people consume in the West. For example, think about the average office worker. He/she might have toast and cereal for breakfast. Mid-morning they may have a biscuit made from wheat. At lunchtime they will grab a sandwich because it's quick and convenient. Mid-afternoon maybe they may eat another

biscuit. During the evening they might eat a pizza or have a pasta dish. OK, this is an extreme example however, it serves to illustrate just how prominent wheat often features in the diet. It's likely to be this repeated exposure that leads to the development of a sensitivity.

Question: I am intolerant to wheat and diary foods. If I miss them out of my diet for long enough, will I be able to re-introduce them in the future?

Answer: There is a greater chance of re-introducing a food to which you are intolerant, compared to a food you might be allergic to. Often, if someone is allergic to a food, they must avoid it for life – for example, a person suffering from coeliac disease (an allergy to gluten). But food intolerances sometimes fade when you abstain from eating the offending food for long enough.

Question: I am doing well with my wheat-free diet but I find it difficult when I'm out with my family and friends especially when we eat out in a restaurant. Will it really matter if I have a little wheat on those occasions?

Answer: This really depends on the individual. Some people may get away with eating a little wheat on the odd occasion. Nevertheless, if they continue to eat wheat on day two or three, even though it's a small amount, they can then start to experience uncomfortable symptoms again. Others may react quite quickly after eating the wheat on just one occasion. The same applies to all other foods that you may be intolerant towards.

Question: Why do so many people who suffer from a grain or dairy intolerance experience Irritable Bowel Syndrome (IBS)?

Answer: Because intolerance to such foods causes irritation or inflammation to the lining of the digestive system. The body's way of dealing with the irritant (food) is to evacuate it from the system as quickly as possible to minimise the length of time that the body is exposed to the allergen. When the offending food is eliminated from the diet for long enough, the digestive system begins to heal and the IBS symptoms often diminish and disappear entirely. I have witnessed this on several occasions.

Question: When someone tests positive for a food intolerance is it absolutely necessary to exclude it from the diet 100%?
Answer: The short answer to that question is yes! To give you an example, I once advised someone who tested positive to wheat to exclude it from his diet for an initial period of four weeks so that we could evaluate the results. This person was suffering from bloating and indigestion but he had high hopes of curing his condition. For the first two weeks he noticed some big improvements. His indigestion and bloating disappeared and he lost eight pounds in weight. Needless to say he was delighted. Unfortunately, during the following two weeks he began to experience a return of symptoms. I asked him to keep a food diary. This revealed that he had been eating the occasional biscuit during his morning break at work –the 'spanner in the works', so to speak. He then missed out the biscuits and began to achieve the same positive results he'd experienced at the start of the programme.

Question: Before beginning my gluten-free diet, I was two stone overweight and seriously lacking in energy. I found that I could put on weight very easily and would watch my calorie intake. Despite this I was unable to shift the extra weight.

Since missing out the gluten-grains, not only have I lost weight, but I also find my appetite has improved and that I can eat larger quantities of foods without putting on the pounds. Why is this?

Answer: In addition to the fact that your body no longer retains excess water because you've avoided eating gluten, your digestion has become much more efficient since it's no longer hampered by the damaging effects of gluten.

Question: Don't people who are intolerant to grains lack fibre in their diet?

Answer: Not if they include the grains they are allowed in whole grain form. Whole grains contain all of the goodness of the grain with nothing removed. For example, brown rice has lots of fibre compared to white rice, which is seriously lacking in fibre. The same can be said of the other gluten-free grains in their whole grain form such as buckwheat (no relation to wheat despite the name), quinoa (a South American grain, see page 27), corn and millet. By consuming these grains you will be getting plenty of fibre in your diet. Also, eating whole grains helps you to regulate your weight. This is because the carbohydrates they contain are slowly converted to sugar for energy due to the presence of the fibre, which slows down the conversion process. The opposite is true with refined grains such as white rice.

4

Gluten intolerance

People who are allergic to gluten are said to suffer from coeliac disease. However, as I explained in the previous chapter, an allergy is very different to an intolerance. A person who suffers from coeliac disease will react very quickly to a small amount of gluten. Conversely, someone who has an intolerance to gluten may not even notice any problems until hours or even one to three days later. In fact over the years I soon learned that there are many different shades of gluten intolerance. For instance, some sufferers may be able to eat bread and/or pasta for, let's say, two days but by day three it begins to adversely affect them. Unfortunately, most doctors are unaware of this situation since they have only been trained to focus upon gluten allergy.

How a gluten-sensitivity can affect you
Once an individual becomes sensitive to gluten the body regards it as a toxin. As previously stated, if you are allergic to gluten the body reacts to the toxin more quickly compared to a gluten intolerance. However, in both cases I believe that

gluten causes damage to the digestive system, including inflammation and irritation, particularly to the lining of the small intestine. Since many nutrients are absorbed through the small intestine, it's easy to see why a gluten allergy or intolerance can result in vitamin and mineral deficiencies. Moreover, my experience in dealing with many gluten-sensitive people over the years has led me to conclude that an inability to lose excess weight is often related to the adverse effect that gluten can have on the body's metabolism.

In the beginning I used to think that the effects of gluten were confined to the digestive system. This proved to be very far from the truth. In fact, over the years I soon realised that the effects of a gluten-sensitivity can manifest themselves in any part of the body, including the following:

- Skin problems
- Arthritis
- Menstrual problems
- Weight gain
- Depression
- Poor attention span
- Headaches
- Migraines
- Fatigue
- Drowsiness
- Mouth ulcers
- Constipation
- Irritable Bowel Syndrome (IBS)
- Flatulence and bloating
- Indigestion
- Acid reflux
- Stomach pain
- Recurrent infections
- Mucous congestion including sinus problems

Incredibly, as with the list of conditions associated with general intolerance on page 18, this list is far from being exhaustive and I continuously encounter new health conditions that respond to a diet free of gluten.

Avoiding gluten

As I explained in the previous chapter, gluten is a type of protein found in wheat, barley, rye and oats. So, if you are gluten-sensitive, you must avoid these foods and any products made from them. Even though some gluten-sensitive people can tolerate oats, my advice would be to omit them from the diet initially to err on the side of caution. The following is a list of foods containing gluten:

- Bread
- Rye bread and pumpernickel
- Spelt (a type of wheat)
- Barley
- Oats
- Alcoholic beverages – beers and some spirits such as grain-based vodka
- Biscuits and cookies
- Pretzels
- Muffins
- Pastry
- Scones
- Couscous
- Durham wheat (mostly in pasta)
- Pasta, macaroni, spaghetti
- Noodles
- Pizza
- Breadcrumb-coated foods such as chicken nuggets and fish fingers
- Bulgar wheat
- Wheat, oat or rye crispbreads
- Yorkshire puddings
- Pancakes
- Semolina
- Stuffings
- Rusks
- Wheat-based breakfast cereals or cereals that include wheat
- Malt or malt extract
- Soy sauce
- Modified wheat starch
- Wheatgerm
- Malt vinegar

The following foods may contain hidden gluten:

- Liquorice
- Confectionery (some chocolate, candy, etc.)
- Stock cubes
- Curry powder
- Sauce mixes
- Gravy powder
- Chips/fries (some may have a wheat coating)
- Sausages
- Soups (some use wheat flour as a thickener)
- Crisps (some include wheat or modified wheat starch)
- Mustard powder

And the good news?

Having looked at the lists above you might be forgiven for asking the question: 'What on earth *can* I eat?' Well, the good news is that there are gluten-free alternatives for many of the items listed. For example, you can purchase gluten-free gravy mix, stock cubes, gluten-free sausages, pasta, biscuits, cereals and flour. The other day I even came across some gluten-free beer in a major supermarket. The range of products is constantly growing, which is good for the gluten-sensitive consumer.

For those who wish to bake their own gluten-free products there are a number of flour substitutes now available. The plain type is usually made from a combination of potato, rice, maize and buckwheat flours. Some manufacturers offer a choice between brown or white gluten-free flour. The brown version is nutritionally superior because it contains fibre as well as more vitamins and minerals.

Individual flours

Rice flour has quite a bland taste but it is a plain flour that can be used to make bread or other bakery products. It can also be used as a thickener.

Chickpea flour is sometimes referred to as gram flour. It is commonly used in Asian cookery – for example, to make bhajis.

Potato flour has a fine texture. It can help to introduce moisture to baked goods.

Cornflour is sometimes mixed with other flours to provide a smooth texture.

Soy flour has a strong taste but can be used sparingly when mixed with other flours. Like potato flour, it adds moisture to baked goods.

Amaranth is made from a grain of the same name and is often added to other flours.

Quinoa (pronounced keen-wah) is a South-American grain that can be used to make baked products. Quinoa flakes are derived from quinoa grains, much as oat flakes are made from oats. They are usually cooked in water and differ from the grains in that they cook more quickly and can be used, for example, to make millet porridge.

Buckwheat flour is not related to wheat despite the name. It is sometimes used to make pancakes, which are popular in the USA.

Gluten-free foods

In addition to the gluten-free products already listed, many other foods are naturally free from gluten. These include meat, fish, dairy products, nuts and seeds (provided they are unprocessed), pulses (such as beans, peas and lentils), eggs, fruits and vegetables.

Label watch

Because gluten is added to so many products it is really important to get into the habit of reading the list of ingredients on cans and packets. Look out for any of the ingredients listed above: for example, modified wheat starch or malt extract. Don't worry, you'll soon know which to avoid. Many products now have allergy advice on their labels and state clearly whether they're gluten-free.

IMPORTANT

In my view, it's very important to adopt the correct mental approach to succeed on a gluten-free diet. The person who dwells on the foods that they can't have is the one who inevitably falters and falls by the wayside. Conversely, those who focus on the wide range of foods they can have will usually stick to their new lifestyle and ultimately reap the rewards of improved health and often much improved weight regulation.

Gluten-free recipes

Breakfast

I always advise people to eat breakfast in order to kick-start their day. This is especially important for anyone who wishes to lose excess weight since the right choice of breakfast can help to regulate blood-sugar levels so you avoid cravings for unhealthy snacks during the day. Also, missing out on breakfast fools your body into thinking that it's being starved and therefore it automatically goes into starvation mode. In other words, your metabolism slows down to conserve calories. This is not good news for those who are prone to weight problems.

Many people diagnosed with a gluten-intolerance are confused about what to eat for breakfast. This isn't surprising when you consider that so many breakfast products are based on wheat and oats. However, there are several gluten-free grain alternatives that can form the basis of a sustaining breakfast. It's also a good idea to choose other foods apart from grains: for example, fruit, yoghurt, nuts and seeds.

Please note: Some of these breakfast ideas include the use of gluten-free bread. If you own a bread-maker you can quite easily make your own using gluten-free flour. However, it is also possible to purchase gluten-free bread. In my experience the best breads are available from specialist health food shops but making your own bread at home is certainly less expensive.

Quinoa Porridge
Serves 1–2

150g/5oz quinoa flakes
175ml/6 fl oz water
50ml/2 fl oz freshly pressed apple or pear juice
¼ tsp ground mixed sweet spice, optional

1 Place the quinoa flakes, water and fruit juice in a medium-sized saucepan. Bring the mixture to the boil, stirring, and then reduce the heat and leave to simmer for about 8 minutes.
2 Turn off the heat, stir in the spice, if desired, and leave to cool before serving.

Gluten-Free muesli
This can be made to your own taste from a mixture of gluten-free flakes, nuts, seeds and dried fruits. You can purchase the grains from a health food shop. Simply place all of the ingredients in a resealable plastic container and mix well. Serve yourself the quantity you desire for breakfast and soak with cow's or goat's milk. If you prefer you can use soya or rice milk. Sweeten with a little honey or brown sugar, if desired.

Examples of ingredients

- Buckwheat flakes
- Rice flakes
- Quinoa flakes
- Millet flakes
- Soya flakes
- Sesame seeds

- Chopped apricots
- Raisins
- Sunflower seeds
- Chopped dates
- Hazelnuts
- Cashew nuts

Rice Cakes with Nut or Seed Butter
Serves 1–2

4 rice cakes
nut or seed butter of your choice (e.g. sunflower, cashew nut,
    peanut, hazelnut)
alfalfa sprouts, optional

Spread a thin layer of nut or seed butter onto the rice cakes
and garnish with alfalfa sprouts, if desired.

Buckwheat Pancakes
Makes approximately 6 pancakes

125g/4oz/1 cup buckwheat flour
pinch of sea salt
1 tsp gluten-free baking powder
1 tbsp honey, plus extra honey to serve
1 egg, beaten
150ml/5 fl oz/⅔ cup milk
1 tbsp olive oil
maple syrup, to serve

1 Mix the flour, salt, baking powder, honey and salt together
   in a mixing bowl. Add the egg and a little milk and mix to
   form a smooth batter. Add the remaining milk and beat to
   incorporate with the rest of the batter.
2 Heat the oil in a frying pan. Add 2 tablespoons of the
   batter and cook until golden underneath, scraping the
   pancake at the edges so that it doesn't stick. Use a fish slice
   to flip over the pancake and cook the other side until
   golden brown.

3 Turn out onto a warmed plate and stack the pancakes between layers of greaseproof paper as you cook them, keeping them warm in the oven. Serve with maple syrup or honey.

Apricot Yoghurt Crunch
Serves 2

40g/1½oz/1 cup cornflakes with added corn syrup,
    not malt extract
2 medium peaches, thinly sliced (or use canned peaches in fruit
    juice)
2x150g/5oz pots of thick natural yoghurt
2 tbsp clear honey

1 Pour the cornflakes into 2 bowls and layer the sliced peaches on top.
2 Add spoonfuls of yoghurt and drizzle honey over the top.

Muesli Spice
Serves 2

40g/1½oz/1 cup cornflakes
20g/¾oz/½ cup puffed rice
3 tbsp millet flakes
2 tbsp dried mixed fruit
2 tbsp cashew nuts
½ tsp ground mixed spice
2 tsp dark brown sugar or 2tbsp of clear honey
milk or plain natural yoghurt, to serve

Mix all the ingredients in a bowl and add milk or yoghurt and serve.

No-Cook Quick Porridge

Serves 2

This no-cook, gluten-free version of porridge is nutritious and easy to prepare. Simply follow the instructions below and you'll have an instant breakfast meal the next day. The porridge is naturally sweetened as the raisins release their natural sugars into the mixture throughout the night.

75g/3oz/½ cup millet flakes
75g/3oz/½ cup buckwheat flakes
75g/3oz/½ cup rice flakes
2 tbsp mixed dried fruit
300ml/10 fl oz/1¼ cups milk or plain natural yoghurt
¼ tsp cinnamon, optional

1 Place the millet, buckwheat and rice flakes in a bowl with the dried fruit. Mix together well.
2 Stir in the milk or yoghurt. Sprinkle with cinnamon, if desired. Cover the bowl with plastic wrap and refrigerate overnight to soak. Serve the next morning for breakfast.

Banana and Strawberry Smoothie

Serves 2

2 large ripe bananas, peeled
6 fresh strawberries, hulled
500ml/18 fl oz/2 cups milk

Using a blender or smoothie maker, blend all of the ingredients together and serve in 2 glasses.

Raisin and Yoghurt Delight
Serves 1

75g/3oz/½ cup raisins, pre-soaked overnight
1x150g/5oz pot plain natural yoghurt

Add the pre-soaked raisins to the yoghurt and mix well. Spoon into a bowl and serve at once.

Gluten-Free Toasted Sandwich
Serves 1
This is a good alternative to toasted sandwiches made from wheat, especially as gluten-free bread is often better toasted.

2 slices gluten-free bread
a little butter or margarine
a little nut or seed butter (e.g. sunflower seed spread)

1 Spread each slice of bread with a little butter or margarine.
2 Spread the other side of each slice of bread with the nut or seed butter, form into a sandwich with the buttered side facing outwards and place in a sandwich-maker. Remove when fully toasted, about 5 minutes, and serve.

Baked Beans on Gluten-Free Toast

Serves 1

This is an excellent alternative to baked beans on toast made from wheat-based bread. Be careful to choose baked beans that are gluten-free. It's usually best to opt for versions that are made from natural ingredients from your local health food shop, as in my experience these are less likely to contain gluten. However, ensure that you check all ingredients carefully.

½ large can of baked beans (220g/8oz)
2 slices gluten-free bread
a little butter or margarine, optional

1 Gently heat the beans in a saucepan, stirring occasionally. Meanwhile, toast the bread in a toaster until golden on both sides.
2 Spread the toast with a thin layer of butter or margarine and transfer to a plate. Pour the heated beans over the toast and serve.

Peach and Banana Milkshake

Serves 1

This is a great early morning energy-booster. You can substitute soya milk or rice milk for cow's milk, if preferred.

1 peach, stoned and sliced (or use canned peaches sweetened in fruit juice)
1 large banana, sliced
500ml/18 fl oz/2 cups milk, chilled

Blend the fruit and milk together in a blender and pour into a glass.

Corn Crispbread and Hummus Spread
Serves 1
If preferred, you can substitute toasted gluten-free bread or rice cakes for the corn crispbread.

2 corn crispbreads
50g/2oz hummus

Spread the hummus over the corn crispbreads and serve.

Scrambled Eggs on Gluten-Free Toast
Serves 2

3 medium eggs
2 tbsp milk
a pinch of sea salt
freshly ground black pepper
½ tbsp butter
4 slices gluten-free bread, spread with a little
    butter or margarine

1 In a bowl, whisk together the eggs, milk and seasoning.
2 Melt the butter gently in a non-stick saucepan over low heat and pour in the scrambled egg mixture.
3 Gently heat and stir until scrambled, about 2–3 minutes depending on how you like your eggs. Place the bread on serving plates, pile scrambled eggs on top and serve.

Fresh Fruit Salad and Fromage Frais
Serves 1
A light and refreshing breakfast – the tangy flavours of the fruit contrast nicely with the fromage frais.

1 breakfast bowl of your favourite fresh fruit, sliced
1 small (150g/5oz) pot fromage frais
1 tbsp finely chopped nuts

Layer the sliced fresh fruit into the bowl and pour fromage frais on top. Sprinkle with the chopped nuts and serve.

Main meals
I encounter many people who test positive for gluten intolerance. Their first reaction is usually one of horror at the prospect of a gluten-free diet. 'But what can I eat?' is a common question. As you'll see from the following recipes, gluten-free doesn't have to be boring. Take a look at these delicious gluten-free meals, and I think you'll agree.

Mediterranean Rice
Serves 4

1 tbsp extra virgin olive oil
1 medium onion, chopped
1 garlic clove, crushed
½ tsp mixed dried herbs
300ml/10 fl oz/1¼ cups water
50g/2oz/⅓ cup red or green pepper, deseeded and chopped
115g/4oz tomatoes, peeled and chopped
125g/4½oz/¾ cup long-grain rice

1 Gently heat the oil in a frying pan and sauté the onion, garlic, mixed herbs and pepper until tender.
2 Stir in the water, pepper, tomatoes and rice. Cover and simmer for around 25 minutes or until the rice is cooked (see package instructions), stirring occasionally. Fluff up with a fork and serve.

Vegetable and Cod Stir-Fry
Serves 2

2 tbsp extra virgin olive oil
1 medium onion, sliced
150g/5oz/1¼ cups carrots, chopped
1 red pepper, deseeded and sliced
1 medium courgette, chopped
1 medium potato, peeled and sliced
25g/8oz cod fillet, skinned and sliced into small pieces
1 tbsp tamari (wheat-free soy) sauce
1 tsp cornflour
50ml/2 fl oz/¼ cup water

1 Warm a wok and heat the oil. Gently stir-fry the vegetables for 5–7 minutes.
2 Add the cod to the wok and stir-fry until the fish is thoroughly cooked, about 8–10 minutes.
3 In a bowl, mix together the tamari sauce, cornflour and water to form a smooth paste. Pour the mixture into the wok and stir into the vegetables. Cook for a further 2 minutes and serve hot.

Baked Sweet Potatoes with Tuna and Vegetables
Serves 2

2 large sweet potatoes
1 tbsp extra virgin olive oil
2 beef tomatoes, finely chopped
1 medium red onion, finely chopped
1 tbsp clear honey
2 tbsp lemon juice
115g/4oz canned tuna in oil or brine
small handful chopped fresh basil
½ tsp sea salt

1 Preheat the oven to 200°C/400°F/Gas 6. Meanwhile, scrub
   the potatoes, prick with a fork and place in a roasting tin
   or dish. Coat with oil and seasoning then bake for around
   40 minutes or until tender.
2 Meanwhile, place tomatoes and onion in a mixing bowl
   and combine with the honey and lemon juice. Stir in the
   tuna, basil and sea salt. Set aside in a cool place.
3 Slice the potatoes in two, quickly scoop out the flesh and
   use a fork to mix in the tuna until combined and fluffy.
4 Fill the scooped-out potatoes with the mixture and serve.

Gluten-Free Pizza with Roasted Vegetables
Serves 4
You can also buy ready-made gluten-free pizza bases for use
with the topping in this recipe.

25g/8oz/2 cups gluten-free flour
¼ tsp sea salt

1 tbsp fresh baker's yeast

1 medium egg

warm water

4 garlic cloves, peeled and sliced lengthways

1 medium courgette, thinly sliced

25g/1oz/⅓ cup mushrooms, sliced

1 tbsp mixed Mediterranean dried herbs

3 tbsp extra virgin olive oil, plus extra to grease

2 tbsp sun-dried tomato paste

65g/2½oz Parmesan cheese, grated

freshly ground black pepper

a little grated carrot, tomatoes and sliced onion, to serve

coriander sprigs, to garnish

salad dressing, to serve

1 Preheat the oven to 200°C/400°F/Gas 6. Meanwhile, sift the flour and seasoning into a bowl. Crumble the yeast and add to the mixture

2 In a separate bowl, beat the egg with about 50ml/ 4 tablespoons/¼ cup water and add to the flour mixture. Knead into a stiff dough, cover and leave to rise in a warm environment.

3 Place the garlic and vegetables on a baking tray, sprinkle with herbs and oil. Bake for approximately 30 minutes until roasted.

4 Roll the dough out into a round pizza shape and place in an oiled ovenproof pizza dish. Spread sun-dried tomato paste on top and layer with roasted vegetables. Sprinkle with Parmesan cheese and bake for a further 20 minutes until the base is properly cooked and the cheese has melted. Grind black pepper over the top and serve.

5 Place the grated carrot in a serving dish and arrange the

tomatoes and onion over the top. Sprinkle with coriander and drizzle with salad dressing. Serve with the pizza.

Cream of Mushroom Soup
Serves 4

oil for frying
225g/8oz/2 cups mushrooms, chopped
300ml/10 fl oz/1¼ cups whole milk
300ml/10 fl oz/1¼ cups gluten-free vegetable stock
50g/2oz cornflour
50g/2oz butter
1 bay leaf
sea salt and freshly ground black pepper
2 tbsp lemon juice
toasted gluten-free bread, to serve

1 Coat a heavy-based frying pan with a little oil. Heat the oil and add the chopped mushrooms. Blend in the milk, stock and cornflour.
2 Place the butter in a separate pan and heat gently until melted. Pour in the blended stock and add the bay leaf. Heat, constantly stirring until the mixture thickens to a smooth consistency.
3 Add the mushrooms to the mixture, remove the bay leaf and blend once more with the seasoning and lemon juice. Serve with slices of toasted gluten-free bread.

Potato and Onion Drop Scones
Makes 10

450g/1lb large potatoes, peeled and cut into small chunks
¼ tsp gluten-free baking powder
2 medium eggs
¼ tsp sea salt
freshly ground black pepper
75ml/3 fl oz/⅓cup milk
1½ tbsp extra virgin olive oil or rapeseed oil, for frying
1 medium onion, finely chopped
gluten-free baked beans or green beans, to serve

1 Place the potatoes in a pan of salted water. Bring to the boil and leave to simmer for 12–15 minutes. When tender, drain well and mash until smooth.
2 Stir in the baking powder, then add the eggs, seasoning and the milk to thoroughly combine.
3 Meanwhile, heat a little oil in a frying pan and sauté the onion over low heat until softened and golden. Add the onions to the potato mixture and mix well.
4 Heat the remaining oil and drop dessertspoonfuls of the mixture into the pan at evenly spaced intervals.
5 Fry for around 4 minutes, turning the scones once with a fish slice, until golden brown. Serve hot with gluten-free baked beans or green beans, if desired.

'Bangers' and Mash with Baked Beans
Serves 2

1 tbsp extra virgin olive oil
4 gluten-free sausages
1 medium onion, sliced
3 large tomatoes, peeled and chopped
1 tsp tamari sauce, optional
1 large can gluten-free baked beans (approx 450g/1lb)
mashed potato, to serve

1 Heat ½ tbsp oil in a frying pan and gently fry the sausages until thoroughly cooked. Slice each one in half.
2 Add the remaining oil to a non-stick saucepan and sauté the onion for a few minutes.
3 Stir in the tomatoes and fry until softened. Add the sausages and baked beans and heat through. Sprinkle with tamari sauce, if desired. Serve hot with mashed potato.

Chicken Risotto
Serves 4

1 tbsp extra virgin olive oil
1 onion, chopped
375g/12oz cooked chicken pieces
2 garlic cloves, crushed
30g/1¼oz mushrooms
50g/2oz/⅓ cup garden peas
350g/12oz/1¾ cups arborio (risotto) rice
¼ tsp sea salt

freshly ground black pepper
1 litre/1¾ pints gluten-free vegetable stock
green salad, to serve

1 Heat the oil in a large frying pan or wok and gently sauté the onion until softened. Add the chicken, garlic, mushrooms, peas and rice. Add the seasoning and stir.
2 Meanwhile, heat the stock in a saucepan and then simmer gently.
3 Add 200ml stock to the rice and continue to cook gently, stirring, until the liquid is absorbed. Continue to add the stock, 200ml at a time, until the rice is throughly cooked (see package directions).
4 Transfer to serving plates and serve with a green salad.

Millet and Savoury Vegetables
Serves 2–3

225g/8oz millet
750ml/1¼ pints water
a little sea salt
2 tbsp extra virgin olive oil, plus extra to grease
2 carrots, grated
3 sticks of celery
2 courgettes, sliced
1 onion, finely diced
200g/7oz tofu
2 tsp tamari sauce
4 tbsp plain yoghurt

1 Preheat the oven to 180°C/350°F/Gas 4 and lightly oil a casserole dish. Rinse the millet, add to a saucepan and cover with water. Add a pinch of sea salt. Bring to the boil, cover and simmer until all the water has been absorbed.

2 Gently heat the oil in a frying pan and add the vegetables. Sauté for 10–12 minutes until softened and golden.

3 Meanwhile, put the tofu, tamari sauce and yoghurt into a liquidiser and blend together.

4 Mix the millet with the vegetables and add about two-thirds of the tofu mixture, stirring to combine. Pour into the casserole dish and add the remainder of the tofu mixture on top.

5 Bake in the centre of the oven for about 25 minutes until golden brown.

Fish Cakes
Serves 4

225g/8oz potatoes, peeled and diced
sea salt
225g/8oz fish, such as cod or haddock
I egg, beaten
2 tsp tomato purée
I small onion, finely chopped
I tbsp parsley
½ tsp freshly ground black pepper
15g/½oz butter
50g/2oz gluten-free breadcrumbs
I lemon, cut into quarters, to serve
gluten-free baked beans or cooked vegetables such as cabbage or
    broccoli, to serve

1 Place the potatoes in a pan and just cover with water. Add a little salt, bring to the boil and simmer until softened, about 10 minutes.

2 After 10 minutes, add fish to potatoes then simmer for 5 minutes.

3 Meanwhile, in a bowl mix together half the egg, the tomato purée, onion, parsley, a pinch of salt and the pepper.

4 Drain the fish and potatoes; remove the skin and any bones from the fish, then flake.

5 Mash the potatoes with a little butter. Add the fish and egg mixture to the potatoes; mix well. Shape into fishcakes, dip in the remaining beaten egg and coat with breadcrumbs.

6 Lightly fry in a little olive oil for 2–3 minutes on one side until crisp and golden, then turn and cook for a further 2–3 on the other side.

7 Serve with lemon quarters, some gluten-free baked beans or some cooked vegetables and new potatoes, if desired.

Mediterranean Roasted Vegetables
Serves 4
This recipe makes a great accompaniment to lightly seasoned cooked rice.

oil, for greasing
3 red onions, cut into quarters
1 orange or red pepper, deseeded and cut into chunks
1 yellow pepper, deseeded and cut into chunks
6 tomatoes, halved
2 medium courgettes, sliced
1 fennel bulb, roughly sliced
1 aubergine, diced

5 garlic cloves

I tbsp extra virgin olive oil

rosemary sprigs

freshly ground black pepper

1 Preheat the oven to 220°C/425°F/Gas 7. Lightly oil an ovenproof roasting dish. Layer the onions, peppers, tomatoes, courgettes, fennel and aubergine.

2 Place the garlic cloves, unpeeled, in among the vegetables and lightly coat with olive oil. Add a few rosemary sprigs to the vegetables and sprinkle with black pepper.

3 Roast for around 25 minutes, turning the vegetables at the halfway stage.

Salads

Anyone who is gluten-sensitive will find the wide variety of fruits and vegetables available now to be a real lifesaver. Obviously they have the advantage of being naturally gluten-free and can form the foundation of a healthy gluten-free diet. If you are not that keen, maybe it's because you haven't properly explored the many ways in which you can combine them. For example, some people think of salads as being a little dull. If you fall into that category, perhaps you need to get away from the lettuce leaf and tomato image that some people still associate with salad meals. Be adventurous when it comes to trying out fruit and vegetables in different combinations, give them a try! I know lots of people who were slightly 'salad phobic' until they experimented with new ideas. So, if you've never been a fan of fruit and veg, just look at the following recipes with an open mind. You may be surprised how much you enjoy them!

Super-Combi Salad

The good thing about this salad is that there really aren't any rules, except to use only gluten-free ingredients in salad dressings and other flavourings. Take a large salad bowl, simply chop up your favourite vegetables and fruits and throw them into the mix! The following list of ingredients should mean that you're never short of ideas:

- Apples
- Carrots
- Lentils of all kinds
- Lettuce and salad leaves
- Mushrooms
- Beans – green (runner or French), broad beans, etc.
- Asparagus
- Beetroot
- Cauliflower
- Peas
- Cabbage (red and white)
- Celery
- Peppers
- Broccoli
- Cucumber
- Chickpeas
- Chicory
- Spinach
- Tomatoes
- Courgettes
- Watercress
- Salad sprouts –alfalfa, mung beans, radish, etc

Additional ingredients

Once you have your basic mixture, you may like to make your salad more interesting by adding one or more of the following ingredients:

- Different varieties of cheese
- Eggs
- Fish
- Meat – especially chicken
- Nuts
- Seeds – pumpkin, sunflower, etc.
- Gluten-free pasta
- Hummus

Added to your salads, these foods will not only give a wide contrast in flavours and textures, but they also provide a source of complex carbohydrates (e.g. pasta), protein, vitamins, minerals and healthy fats.

Other ingredient

If liked, you can also add some of the following ingredients:

- Olives
- Avocadoes
- Bananas
- Grapes
- Pine nuts
- Raisins

- Oranges
- Coconut
- Pears
- Dates
- Fresh herbs – chopped mint, oregano, etc

Salad dressings

Interesting dressings can make all the difference to a salad. You can make your own or purchase a gluten-free dressing from your local supermarket or health food shop. Healthy gluten-free ingredients include olive oil, cider vinegar, herbs and honey or agave syrup. Agave syrup is derived from a cactus and believe it or not, it is really delicious! Below are some other exciting salad ideas for you to try.

Homemade Coleslaw

Serves 2

Serve with a baked potato, if desired.

¼ white cabbage, grated

1 or 2 carrots, finely grated

1 red pepper, deseeded and chopped

1 tbsp olive oil

1 tbsp natural gluten-free mayonnaise
freshly ground black pepper

1 Place the cabbage in a bowl together with the carrot and red pepper.
2 In another container, whisk together the oil and mayonnaise with a fork.
3 Pour the mixture over the vegetables and stir well.

Grated Carrot and Celeriac with Raisins or Dates
Serves 2

½ celeriac, peeled and grated
2 medium carrots, grated
a handful of dates or raisins
1 tbsp gluten-free mayonnaise or French dressing
gluten-free bread or rice cakes, to serve

Place the celeriac and carrots in a bowl together with the raisins or dates. Pour the dressing over the mixture and stir well to combine. Serve with gluten-free bread or rice cakes.

Brown Rice Salad
Serves 2

150g/5oz/⅞ cup brown rice
300ml/10 fl oz/2 cups water
a little sea salt
1 red or yellow pepper, deseeded and chopped
1 medium red onion, finely diced

75g/3oz/¾ cup broad beans or peas
75g/3oz/¾ cup roasted peanuts (not dry-roasted)
I tbsp raisins or sultanas
gluten-free French dressing, to serve

1 Place the rice in a saucepan with the water. Bring to the boil, reduce the heat and simmer gently until all the water has been absorbed. Add sea salt to taste.
2 Place the cooked rice in a mixing bowl and stir in the vegetables, roasted peanuts and raisins or sultanas. Add dressing to taste, mix well and serve at once.

Finger Salad
Serves 1–2
The salad combines well with rice cakes or corn crispbread spread with a little butter or margarine.

I stick of celery, cut into 2.5cm/Iin batons
I medium carrot, cut into batons
2 spring onions, trimmed
¼ raw cauliflower, cut into bite-size florets
a few cherry tomatoes
gluten-free dip of your choice or hummus, to serve

Serve the prepared vegetables with your favourite gluten-free dip such as mint and yoghurt or a bowl of hummus.

Avocado, Tomato, Iceberg Lettuce and Prawn Salad
Serves 1

50g/2oz/1 cup finely chopped iceberg lettuce
4 tomatoes, sliced
1 ripe avocado, stoned, peeled and sliced
50g/2oz small tub of Icelandic prawns
2 tbsp gluten-free mayonnaise
1 tsp cayenne pepper
gluten-free bread, to serve

1 Arrange the lettuce on a serving plate. Add a layer of tomatoes and sliced avocado.
2 In a bowl, combine the prawns with the mayonnaise and spoon the mixture onto the centre of the salad.
3 Sprinkle with cayenne pepper and serve with slices of gluten-free bread.

Pasta Salad
Serves 2

150g/5oz/⅞ cup gluten-free pasta
2 spring onions, trimmed and finely chopped
1 red and 1 yellow pepper, deseeded and finely sliced
1 small can of sweetcorn, drained and rinsed (approx 200g/7oz)
1 medium courgette, cut into small strips
75g/3oz canned tuna, drained

1 Bring a medium pan of salted water to the boil, add the pasta and cook according to the package directions until

just cooked (al dente). Drain the pasta, refresh in cold water and transfer to a bowl.

2 Add the vegetables and tuna to the pasta; mix well and serve.

Rice and Baked Bean Salad
Serves 1

115g/4oz/¾cup basmati rice
180g/6⅓oz/1 cup chopped cherry tomatoes
1 red onion, diced
1 carrot, grated
a handful of pine nuts
½ small can gluten-free baked beans (approx 200g/7oz)

1 Place the rice in a saucepan with twice its volume of water. Bring to the boil and leave to simmer for 20 minutes. Drain and cool.
2 Transfer to a bowl and add the tomatoes, onion, carrot, pine nuts and baked beans. Mix well and serve.

Cauliflower, Carrot, Beetroot and Chicken Salad
Serves 2

¼ cauliflower, cut into bite-sized pieces
1 beetroot, grated
1 carrot, grated
a handful of sunflower seeds
200g/7oz bite-sized chicken pieces
gluten-free croûtons

your favourite salad dressing
gluten-free bread or rice cakes, to serve

1 Place the cauliflower, beetroot and carrot in a bowl.
2 Add the sunflower seeds, chicken pieces and croûtons.
  Drizzle with salad dressing and mix together well. Serve
  with gluten-free bread or rice cakes.

Carrot, Onion and Tomato Salad
Serves 2

4 tomatoes, sliced
2 medium carrots, grated
I medium red onion, thinly sliced
2 tbsp extra virgin olive oil or cold pressed rapeseed oil
2 tbsp chopped fresh coriander
I tbsp red wine or cider vinegar
I tsp clear honey
freshly ground black pepper
a pinch of sea salt

1 Place the grated carrot in a serving dish and arrange the
  tomatoes and onion over the top.
2 Prepare a dressing by mixing the oil, honey, salt and
  pepper together.
3 Pour over the salad and serve with gluten-free bread or
  rice cakes, if desired.

Desserts

There are a number of gluten-free desserts that you can incorporate into your everyday diet. In addition to the recipes that follow, there are also a number of basic ready-made desserts that you can purchase from supermarkets or health food shops. Some of the ingredients, such as cashew nuts and almond butter, are available from health food shops. They are superior to peanut butter as they contain healthier fats. Consider the options listed below:

Ice cream Look for ice cream with a label stating that it is gluten-free. Ice creams containing natural ingredients are less likely to also include other additions such as modified wheat starch, which you'll need to avoid.

Soya desserts Today there are some very nice soya desserts to choose from. They come in a variety of flavours such as chocolate, strawberry, carob and vanilla. Most are gluten-free, but remember to check the labels.

Soya cream It's now possible to purchase soya cream, which is a delicious alternative to ordinary cream. It makes a great accompaniment to fresh fruit and desserts such as apple crumble.

Carob This ingredient comes from the carob bean that grows in the warm climate of Mediterranean countries such as Spain. The pods have a pleasantly sweet taste and when ground into powder, they are used to make chocolate-like confectionery. Some of the carob bars that you can buy are very tasty and serve as a good alternative to chocolate. However, you'll need to study the list of ingredients carefully because certain brands include wheat, oats or modified wheat starch. Look out for the varieties containing natural ingredients such as coconut and dried fruit.

Real custard Packets of natural custard are available from health food shops. They're usually based on cornflour, which is free from gluten. Again, always check the ingredients label.

Sorbets Most commercially produced sorbets are usually free from gluten, but some may contain modified starch, so just be careful. You can make them easily at home using natural fruit juices, or squeezed lemon juice and a natural sweetener such as clear honey or agave syrup (see page xx).

Ice lollies These are simple to make using natural fruit juices which you pour into a lolly mould and place in the freezer. There are plenty of juices to choose from, including pineapple, apple, orange, grape, and the more exotic juices such as kiwi and mango. The good news is that they're all naturally gluten-free!

Fresh fruit and bio-yoghurt Another naturally good, gluten-free option. The slightly sour flavour of the natural yoghurt makes a great combination with sweet, succulent fruits such as kiwi, grapes, melon, apple and pear.

Baked Bananas
Serves 2

3 tbsp lemon or orange juice
1 tsp Muscovado sugar
3 tbsp dried fruit
3 large bananas
½ tsp cinnamon powder
1 small pot plain natural yoghurt (approx 150g/5oz) or ice cream, to serve

1 Preheat the oven to 180°C/350°F/Gas 4. Meanwhile, combine the citrus juice, sugar and dried fruit in a small bowl.

2 Arrange each of the bananas on a square of foil and carefully pour over the mixture. Sprinkle with cinnamon. Wrap each banana in foil to form a parcel, place on a baking tray and warm through for 12–15 minutes. Serve with yoghurt or ice cream.

Fruit Muffins
Makes 12

225g/8oz/2 cups gluten-free plain flour
a pinch of sea salt
30g/1¼oz Muscovado sugar
I tsp gluten-free baking powder
50ml/2floz/¼cup milk
2 tbsp rapeseed or olive oil
I medium egg, beaten
75g/3oz mixed vine fruit (dried raisins, sultanas and currants)

1 Preheat the oven to 220°C/425°F/Gas 7. Meanwhile, mix the flour, salt, sugar and baking powder together in a bowl. Combine the milk, oil, egg and dried fruit.

2 Place 12 muffin cases onto a baking tray and divide the mixture between them. Bake in the centre of the oven for 12–15 minutes until risen and golden. Cool on a wire rack.

Blackberry and Apple Crumble
Serves 4

450g/1 lb Bramley or other cooking apples, peeled, cored and
  quartered
225g/8oz blackberries
25ml/1 fl oz water
115g/4oz/¾ cup light brown sugar, plus extra for
  sprinkling, if desired
¾ tsp ground mixed spice
50g/2oz/½ cup rice flour
50g/2oz/½ cup potato flour
50g/2oz butter
soya cream, to serve (optional)

1 Preheat the oven to 180°C/350°F/Gas 4. Arrange the apples
   and blackberries in an ovenproof dish and sprinkle with
   water and half the sugar. Then sprinkle with spice.
2 Sieve the flours in to a bowl, add the butter and rub in with
   your fingertips until the mixture forms a crumbly texture.
   Add the remaining sugar and mix well.
3 Layer the crumble evenly over the apples and blackberries
   and press down lightly. Sprinkle with a little extra sugar, if
   desired, for a crunchy texture.
4 Bake in the centre of the oven for approximately 40–50
   minutes until the crumble is a golden colour. Serve warm
   with soya cream, if desired.

Sweet Buckwheat Pancakes
Serves 2

115g/4oz/1½ cups buckwheat flour
a pinch of sea salt
2 eggs
3 tbsp clear honey
250ml/8 fl oz/1 cup whole milk
30g/1¼oz butter, melted
1 tbsp extra virgin olive oil
1 lemon, cut into wedges

1 Preheat the oven to 150°C/300°F/Gas 2. Sift the flour and salt into a bowl and make a well in the centre. Add the eggs, 2 tbsp honey and half the milk. Mix thoroughly to form a thick, smooth batter.
2 Add the remaining milk and the butter; beat for 3 minutes. Leave the mixture to stand for about 30 minutes.
3 Pour the olive oil into a non-stick frying pan and heat to a high temperature. Add enough batter to cover the base and swirl it around to coat evenly. When the edges of the pancake begin to brown, use a fish slice to flip it over and cook until golden brown on the other side.
4 Keep the pancake warm on a plate in the oven while you cooking the remaining pancakes (stack between layers of greaseproof paper). Drizzle with the remaining honey and serve with the lemon wedges.

Tropical Fruit Salad and Thick Greek Yoghurt
Serves 2

2 kiwi fruits, peeled and cut into slices
¼ fresh pineapple, peeled and cut into chunks
5 apricots, cut into quarters
12 red seedless grapes, halved
1 small mango, de-seeded and cut into small chunks
150ml/5 fl oz thick Greek yoghurt
1 tbsp clear honey or agave syrup (see page 49)

Divide the fruit between serving bowls. Layer an equal amount of yoghurt over each bowl and drizzle honey or agave syrup on top.

Healthy gluten-free snacks

If you have a problem with gluten, it's really important that you carry some healthy gluten-free snacks with you at all times. If you select healthy snacks that don't cause significant fluctuations in your blood sugar levels, you'll be more in control of your weight as well as your energy levels. There are lots of gluten-free options but it's essential that the snacks are healthy too because unhealthy snacks just give you a quick burst of energy followed by a slump. When this happens you simply crave more snacks and that's the time when you're most likely to be tempted by foods containing gluten. The following snacks are naturally gluten-free:

Fresh fruit Choose apples, pears, kiwi, pineapple, oranges, peaches, grapes, melon, bananas or whatever is in season.
Dried fruit Look for unsulphured and preservative-free

raisins, sultanas, dates, figs, apricots and currents. It is preferable to ingest fruit not subjected to sulphur dioxide gas, used to bleach dried fruits. Dried fruits are a good source of vitamins and minerals but eat them in moderation because they are high in fruit sugar and can be fattening if you have too many.

Popcorn Corn can be a good option since it doesn't contain gluten. Homemade popcorn is easily prepared and much healthier than commercial types! Cook the corn in a frying pan or skillet in a little olive oil and use a little sea salt or a natural sweetener such as fructose (fruit sugar) in small amounts.

Crudités Use raw vegetables such as carrots, courgettes, celery, cucumber and cauliflower cut into bite-size pieces. They are delicious with a tasty dip such as hummus or gluten-free mayonnaise.

Rice cakes These are a bit like Marmite, you either love them or hate them! I find that what makes the difference is what you spread over them. For example, rice cakes can be delicious spread with hummus, gluten-free pâté or honey if you want something sweet.

Corn crispbreads Similar to rice cakes, but made from corn.

Ready-made gluten-free snacks You can purchase items such as gluten-free fruit bars from health food shops and some supermarkets.

Nuts Always a good energy sustaining snack. Avoid processed nuts such as dry-roasted peanuts as they may contain gluten. Unsalted, raw (not roasted) nuts are always the best option. Choose from cashews, hazelnuts, pine nuts, walnuts, pecans, almonds, Brazil nuts, etc. Nuts and raisins are also a good combination, but do eat nuts in moderation as they are high in calories.

Seeds Avoid processed seeds, especially those flavoured with soya sauce or any other ingredient containing gluten. Choose from sunflower, pumpkin and sesame. Hemp seeds are also a great-tasting option, but make sure you select the hulled type as the others are a bit crunchy.

Suzanne's story

I decided to take the test because I thought I had a sensitivity to wheat; I felt bloated and tired when I ate wheat bread so tried to eat alternatives such as rye bread and oat cakes. However, the test showed that I had a gluten intolerance and should avoid not just wheat but oats, barley and rye! If I hadn't have taken the test I would never have realised this.

Immediately after the test I embarked on a gluten-free diet. For two days I had a mild headache but after this I immediately noticed a difference. My bloated stomach had gone down and I had significantly more energy – getting out of bed in the morning wasn't such a struggle and doing physical tasks around the house didn't feel so onerous – I was even doing my ironing at 6.30am one morning!

After one month on a gluten-free diet I have lost 9lb, which I'd had difficulty shifting before. I don't get the cravings for wheat-based foods such as bread, cakes and biscuits which I use to get, especially when I was stressed with work. This means I am more in control of my eating habits and I don't over eat or eat the wrong foods as I am absorbing the nutrients more efficiently from the food I eat. My diet is therefore much healthier and I feel better.

I am delighted with the results and have recommended the test to family and friends as it has significantly changed my life. I am currently training for a 26-mile charity walk and have more energy. Feeling more positive means I can fit the training into a busy daily schedule, which involves running my own business and caring for a young son.

5

Wheat intolerance

As with gluten, you can be either allergic or intolerant to wheat. My experience in this field has taught me that sensitivity to wheat is amazingly common. In fact, I would go further and say that it has reached almost epidemic proportions. People often ask me why it's such a big problem these days. Personally, I feel that it's down to a number of factors, including the fact that we in the West consume so much wheat on a daily basis. In reality, our so-called Western-style of diet contains an amazing amount of wheat-based products. The end result is that our bodies are bombarded with wheat on a daily basis.

Most authorities on the subject of allergies and food intolerances are aware that constant over-exposure to one food type can increase one's propensity to develop sensitivity to that food. This has certainly been borne out of my experience with food intolerance testing. Unbelievably, I'm finding that as many as five out of ten people who are tested have a problem with wheat. Other reasons why wheat causes so many problems may include the increasing use of chemicals such as pesticides and fungicides in the growing process. Additionally, in evolutionary terms grains have only been included in our diet for a relatively short time. Prior to this our prehistoric ancestors appeared to have lived on a diet consisting mostly of fruits, some vegetables, nuts, seeds and perhaps a little meat or fish depending on their geographical location. In essence, this means we just haven't had time to adapt to grains and hence the reason why they are known to be one of the food groups most likely to evoke an allergic response.

Symptoms connected to wheat intolerance

As with gluten sensitivity, wheat allergy and wheat intolerance can result in a wide range of health conditions including arthritis, headaches, migraines, menstrual irregularities, mouth ulcers, recurrent infections, mucous congestion, sinus pain, watery and itchy eyes, runny nose, eczema and other skin conditions, low energy, drowsiness, muscle pain, mood swings, depression, constipation, Irritable Bowel Syndrome (IBS), indigestion, bloating, stomach pains, acid reflux, poor absorption of nutrients and of course, as you'll now be aware, an inability to lose excess weight. If you are following a wheat-free diet, here is a list of foods to avoid:

- Bread made with wheat flour (including chappatis, naan, pitta, tortillas and some rye breads with added wheat). Always check the labels
- Breakfast cereals made with wheat and those with added wheat such as most mueslis
- Beer
- Pasta, macaroni and spaghetti
- Noodles
- Bulgar wheat
- Durhum wheat

- Pizza
- Scones
- Cakes and muffins
- Anything made with breadcrumbs
- Anything in batter (or made of batter, such as pancakes)
- Semolina
- Pretzels
- Biscuits made with wheat flour
- Pastry
- Stuffings
- Wheat bran and wheat flours, including spelt
- Wheatgerm
- Wheat noodles
- Cereal binders
- Citric acid (some brands may have been made with wheat)
- Dextrins (some contain wheat)
- Farina
- Ground spices (always check the ingredients label)
- Mustard powder
- Packets of shredded suet
- Edible starch (this may be made from wheat)
- Soy sauce
- Stock cubes (some may contain wheat so check the ingredients list)
- Gum base

As with gluten intolerance, it pays to scrutinise labels. Obviously if a product says wheat-free, then that's fine. However, remember that a gluten-free product must be wheat-free too. It's also important to note that a wheat-free diet can include rye, barley and oats unlike a gluten-free diet so this gives you more scope when it comes to alternative options to wheat.

Wheat-free recipes

Some of the following recipes contain ingredients such as oats, barley and rye. Where the use of flour is required, gluten-free or wheat-free flour may be included in the recipe.

Breakfast

Banana-Hazelnut Delight
Serves 1

1 large banana
1 small pot (approx 150g/5oz) thick Greek yoghurt
1 tsp clear honey
1 tbsp chopped hazelnuts (or substitute your favourite nuts)
¼ tsp cinnamon
2 slices wheat-free rye bread, toasted

In a bowl, mash the banana with a fork and mix in the yoghurt and honey. Fold in the nuts and serve with the rye bread toast.

No-Cook Porridge
Serves 1
This is a quick, no-cook breakfast for people in a hurry as it can be prepared the night before. No added sugar is required because the natural sugars in the fruit permeate the oats and milk overnight. However, a little honey or agave syrup (see page 49) can be added, if extra sweetness is desired.

150g/5oz/1 cup oat flakes
2 tbsp sultanas
a pinch of cinnamon
150ml/5 fl oz semi-skimmed milk

1 Pour the oats into a breakfast bowl. Add the sultanas and
   cinnamon and mix together to combine.
2 Pour the milk onto the mixture and stir.
3 Cover the bowl with plastic wrap and refrigerate overnight.
   Enjoy as a quick and nutritious breakfast in the morning.

Tahini on Rye
Serves 1
Quick and easy to prepare. Tahini is a spread made from
sesame seeds and a good source of healthy fats.

2 slices rye bread made from 100% rye
40g/1½oz tahini spread
a little butter or margarine
freshly squeezed juice, to serve

Toast the rye bread and spread with a thin layer of butter or
margarine, followed by the tahini spread. Serve with a freshly
squeezed juice such as orange or grapefruit.

Fruity Oatcakes and Bio-Yoghurt
Serves 1
The jam used in this recipe is sweetened with concentrated
fruit juice and not cane sugar, which is a healthy alternative
to ordinary jam. It is available in most supermarkets and

health food shops. The bio-yoghurt is so-called because it contains beneficial bacteria that promote a healthy digestive system. The sour taste of the yoghurt complements the sweetness of the jam perfectly.

3–4 oatcakes made from 100% oats
a little butter or margarine
about 2 tbsp unsweetened natural jam of your choice
1 small pot (approx 150g/5oz)plain bio-yoghurt

Spread the oatcakes with a thin layer of butter or margarine followed by the jam. Serve with bio-yoghurt on the side.

Oat and Honey Grapefruit Delight
Serves 2

2 tbsp clear honey
1 tbsp raisins
2 tbsp rolled oats
2 large grapefruit, preferably pink for the best flavour
½ tsp ground mixed spice

Preheat the grill to medium. Meanwhile, mix the honey, raisins and oats in a saucepan over a low heat until thoroughly combined. Halve and segment each grapefruit. Top each half with the oat mixture and grill for 4–5 minutes. Sprinkle with sweet spice and serve at once.

'Jammy' Rye Toastie
Serves 1

2 slices 100% rye bread
a little butter
4 tsp jam (choose your favourite variety)
pressed fruit juice, to serve

1 Coat one side of each slice of bread with a thin layer of butter.
2 Spread the jam over the dry side of one of the slices and then, with buttered sides facing outwards, form a sandwich.
3 Place the sandwich in a sandwich toaster and cook until golden brown, for around 5 minutes. Serve with a glass of pressed fruit juice such as apple or orange.

Bio-Yoghurt and Berry Delight
Serves 1
This is a healthy breakfast made from seasonal berries combined with bio-yoghurt, which is a source of healthy bacteria.

75g/3oz/½ cup strawberries (sliced) or raspberries
1 small pot (approx 150g/5oz) plain bio-yoghurt
40g/1½oz/¼ cup blueberries
40g/1½oz/¼ cup blackberries
1 tbsp hulled hempseeds (available from health food shops)
1 tbsp clear honey or agave syrup (see page 49)

1 Rinse the berries and pat dry on kitchen paper.
2 Place the strawberries or raspberries in a breakfast bowl and layer a third of the yoghurt over the top. Repeat the process with the other berries.

3 Sprinkle with the hempseeds then drizzle with honey or agave syrup and serve.

Scrambled Eggs on Rye
Serves 2

a little butter or 1 tbsp extra virgin olive oil
3 medium eggs
3 tbsp milk
a pinch of sea salt and freshly ground black pepper
2 slices 100% rye bread
gluten-free tomato ketchup, to serve, if desired

1 Gently melt the butter or heat the oil in a saucepan.
2 Meanwhile, in a bowl quickly whisk together the eggs, milk and seasoning. Cook over low heat, stirring, until scrambled, depending on how you like your eggs.
3 While the eggs are cooking, toast the rye bread. Pile the scrambled eggs over the toasted bread and serve with tomato ketchup on the side, if desired.

Oatmeal Porridge
Serves 2

150g/5oz/1 cup porridge oats
250ml/8 fl oz/2 cups water or milk
1 tbsp clear honey or agave syrup (see page 49)
a pinch of sea salt
a pinch of grated nutmeg

Place the oats and the water or milk in a saucepan and bring to the boil for 1 minute, stirring constantly. Stir in the honey or syrup, sprinkle with the nutmeg and serve.

Mixed Berry Yoghurt Smoothie

Serves 1

This is a very refreshing breakfast drink. It's also a good energy booster and full of antioxidants.

1 small pot (aprox 150g/5oz) plain bio-yoghurt

65g/2 1/2oz/½ cup mixed berries such as blueberries, blackcurrants, raspberries, hulled if necessary

1 tsp clear honey or agave syrup (see page 49)

½ tsp alcohol-free natural vanilla essence (available from health food shops)

4 ice cubes

Place all of the ingredients in a blender and blend until smooth. Pour into a glass and drink immediately. This is because nutrients and the live enzymes present in the fruit deteriorate the longer they are exposed to the air.

Wheat-Free Muesli

You can make your own wheat-free muesli in much the same way as the gluten-free version in Chapter 4 (see page 30). However, unlike the gluten-free muesli you can also include oats, barley and rye flakes. Simply place your choice of ingredients in a resealable plastic container, mix well and serve with milk or a milk alternative such as soya or rice milk. If you prefer a sweetener, try clear honey or agave syrup (see page 49). Here are some ideas for ingredients that you may wish to combine:

- Buckwheat flakes
- Rice flakes
- Quinoa flakes
- Millet flakes
- Soya flakes
- Sesame seeds
- Chopped apricots
- Raisins
- Sunflower seeds
- Chopped dates
- Hazelnuts
- Cashew nuts
- Oat flakes
- Rye flakes
- Barley flakes
- Hulled hempseeds

Spicy Apple Millet Porridge
Serves 1

25g/1oz millet flakes
200ml/7 fl oz apple juice
1 tsp clear honey or agave syrup (see page 49)
½ tsp ground mixed spice
1 small pot (approx 150g/5oz) plain bio-yoghurt, to serve

1 Place the millet flakes and apple juice in a saucepan and heat gently for 7–8 minutes, stirring frequently until the mixture thickens.
2 Stir in the honey or agave syrup and sprinkle with mixed spice. Serve with the bio-yoghurt.

Soaked Date and Apricot with Fromage Frais
Serves 1
The dates and apricots for this dish should be soaked in water overnight and refrigerated, covered, until required the next morning.

75g/3oz/½ cup pitted dates, soaked overnight
75g/3oz/½ cup unsulphured apricots, soaked overnight
1 small pot (150g/5oz) fromage frais

Drain the dates and apricots and place in a breakfast bowl. Top with fromage frais and serve at once.

Main meals
As you'll see from the following recipes, there is a huge amount of variety if you are following a wheat-free diet.

Butternut and Potato Curry
Serves 4

2 tsp olive oil
1 onion, roughly chopped
2 garlic cloves, crushed
450g/1lb butternut squash, deseeded and cut into chunks
450g/1lb potatoes, cut into chunks
1 cooking apple, cored and cut into chunks
2 tsp medium or mild wheat-free curry paste
1 small piece of fresh root ginger, peeled and finely chopped
2 bay leaves
50g/2oz sultanas
500ml/18 fl oz/3 cups wheat-free vegetable stock

I tsp turmeric
¼ tsp sea salt
freshly ground black pepper
25ml/1 fl oz coconut cream
brown or white basmati rice, to serve

1 Gently heat the olive oil in a large frying pan and fry the
   onion until golden and softened. Add the garlic, butternut
   squash, potatoes and apple.
2 Stir in the curry paste, ginger, bay leaves, sultanas, stock,
   turmeric and seasoning. Add the creamed coconut and
   stir well.
3 Bring to the boil, then simmer for about 12–15 minutes,
   stirring occasionally, until the vegetables are tender. Serve
   over brown or white basmati rice.

Spicy Falafels and Green Salad
Makes 12 falafels

225g/8oz canned chickpeas or dried chickpeas, soaked overnight
I tbsp chopped fresh parsley
I tsp cumin seeds
½ tsp chilli powder
I tsp ground coriander
I garlic clove, crushed
juice of I lemon
I medium egg
½ tsp sea salt
I tbsp oil, plus extra for drizzling
green salad, to serve

1 Preheat the oven to 220°C/425°F/Gas 7.
2 If using dried chickpeas, drain and place in a saucepan. Cover with water and bring to the boil. Maintain the heat for around 15–20 minutes.
3 Drain the cooked or canned chickpeas and place in a food processor, along the parsley, cumin seeds, chilli powder, coriander, garlic, lemon juice, egg and the seasoning. Blend until finely chopped, but not puréed.
4 Moisten your hands and shape the mixture into 12 balls. Use the oil to grease a baking sheet and arrange the falafels so that they are evenly spaced on top.
5 Drizzle lightly with oil and bake for about 15 minutes until golden brown. Serve on a bed of green salad.

Wheat-Free Spaghetti Bolognese
Serves 2

1 tbsp extra virgin olive oil
1 onion, chopped
1 garlic clove, finely chopped
225g/8oz minced beef
50g/2oz mushrooms, sliced
1 large can tomatoes (approx 400g/14oz)
1 carrot, grated
1 tbsp tomato paste
225ml/8 floz wheat-free vegetable stock (made from a wheat- or gluten-free stock cube and water)
1 tsp oregano
freshly ground black pepper
a pinch of sea salt
cooked wheat-free spaghetti, to serve

1 Pour the olive oil into a large saucepan and heat through.
2 Add the onions and garlic; fry gently for a few minutes until softened and golden.
3 Reduce the heat, stir in the minced beef and continue frying for about 10–12 minutes.
4 Add the remaining ingredients, mix together well and leave to simmer until the sauce is reduced. Serve with wheat-free spaghetti cooked according to the package directions.

Vegetable Stew

Serves 4

2 tbsp extra virgin olive oil
1 onion, chopped
2 garlic cloves, finely chopped
1 green chilli pepper, deseeded and finely sliced
1 red or green pepper, deseeded and sliced
½ medium onion squash (or other squash), cut into
    small chunks
2 courgettes, sliced
75g/3oz/½ cup garden peas
½ small cabbage, chopped
600ml/1 pint wheat or gluten-free vegetable stock
115g/4oz canned, cooked chickpeas, drained
1 large can tomatoes (approx 400g/14oz)
¼ tsp sea salt
freshly ground black pepper

1 Gently heat the oil in a large saucepan. Add the onion, garlic and chilli and fry for about 3 minutes.

2 Add the pepper, squash, courgettes, garden peas or cabbage and fry for a further 10–12 minutes.
3 Stir in the stock, chickpeas and tomatoes; season well and serve.

Baked Fish with Brown Rice
Serves 2

juice of 1 lemon
1 garlic clove, finely chopped
1 tsp wheat-free tamari (soy) sauce
1 whole fish, such as bass, cleaned and pin-boned
115g/4oz/¼ cup wholegrain short grain rice, to serve
a little sea salt

1 Preheat the oven to 200°C/400°F/Gas 6.
2 Mix together the lemon juice, garlic and tamari sauce in a bowl.
3 Place the fish on a square of foil and pour over the sauce. Wrap the fish in the foil and bake in the centre of the oven for 40–45 minutes until thoroughly cooked.
4 Meanwhile, place the rice in a saucepan with a pinch of sea salt. Add twice the volume of water and bring to the boil. Leave to simmer according to the package directions until the rice is soft. Drain and keep warm, and arrange on a serving plate with the fish on top. Serve immediately.

Fish Pie
Serves 4

450g/1lb potatoes, chopped
450g/1lb cod or other fish
25g/8oz/2½ cups garden peas
1 medium carrot, sliced
25g butter or margarine
1 tbsp wheat-free or gluten-free flour
150ml/¼ pint/¾ cup skimmed milk, plus a little extra for mashing the
  potatoes
¼ tsp sea salt
a pinch of freshly ground black pepper

1 Place the potatoes in a saucepan and cover with salted water. Bring to the boil and then reduce the heat to simmer until cooked, about 15–20 minutes.
2 Meanwhile, place the fish in a frying pan with just enough water to cover and poach for 5–6 minutes. While the fish is poaching, cook the peas and carrot in a saucepan with just enough boiling salted water to cover. Simmer until tender, then drain.
3 Drain the fish and remove the skin and any bones carefully.
4 Preheat the grill to medium-high. Meanwhile, place half the butter or margarine in a small saucepan and stir in the flour over a low heat to form a thick paste. Gradually add the milk, stirring, to create a smooth white sauce. Keep warm.
5 Arrange the fish, carrots and peas in a large ovenproof dish. Pour over the hot sauce and keep warm under the grill.
6 Drain and mash the potatoes with a little skimmed milk, season and spread them over the fish. Dot with butter then return to the grill to brown and serve.

Vegetable Soup
Serves 4

2 tbsp oil
2 medium onions, finely chopped
1 leek, trimmed and thinly sliced
¼ cauliflower, chopped
2 courgettes, sliced
2 carrots, sliced
1 litre/13/4 pints/5 cups wheat-free vegetable stock
1 tsp mixed herbs
½ large can cooked lentils (225g/8oz)
¼ tsp sea salt
a little pepper
rye or wheat-free bread, to serve

1 Gently heat the oil in a large saucepan and fry the onions until softened and golden. Add the leek, cauliflower, courgettes and carrots and fry for 10–12 minutes.
2 Stir the stock into the mixture and add the herbs, lentils and seasoning. Bring to the boil and then reduce the heat and simmer for about 20 minutes, stirring occasionally.
3 Serve with rye or wheat-free bread.

Vegetable Chilli
Serves 4

1 large can cooked red kidney beans, drained and rinsed (approx 450g/1lb)
1 small can of sweetcorn, drained and rinsed (approx 250g/8oz)
1 large can chopped tomatoes (approx 450g/1lb)

2 courgettes, sliced
I onion, chopped
I I5g/4oz/I¼ cups garden peas
I garlic clove, chopped
I tbsp wheat-free tamari sauce.
I beef tomato, chopped
I tbsp chopped fresh basil
I tsp chilli powder
300g/I0oz/2½ cups brown or white rice

1 Preheat the oven to 180°C/350°F/Gas 4. Place all the
  ingredients except the rice into a large ovenproof casserole
  dish and mix together well. Bake for around 40 minutes.
2 Meanwhile, cook the rice according to the package
  directions and when ready, serve with the casserole.

Spanish Omelette
Serves 2
Serve with your favourite cooked vegetables or with a salad of
green leaves and sliced tomatoes, if desired.

I tbsp extra virgin olive oil
I large onion, thinly sliced
I courgette, sliced
50g/2oz/½ cup mushrooms, sliced
200g/7oz/I cup cooked wholegrain rice or wheat-free pasta
2 large tomatoes, chopped
4 medium eggs
a pinch of sea salt
freshly ground black pepper

1 Preheat the grill to high. Meanwhile, heat half the oil in a large, heavy-based frying pan and add the onion, courgette, mushrooms and rice or pasta. Gently fry for 4–5 minutes.

2 Add the tomatoes and cook for a further 2–3 minutes.

3 Meanwhile, beat the eggs in a bowl and season with salt and pepper.

4 Add the remaining oil to the frying pan and spread the contents evenly over the surface. Pour in the beaten egg mixture.

5 Cook over a medium heat until the omelette is set, scraping to loosen the sides and ensure all the egg is cooked. Finish by browning the omelette slightly under the grill while still in the pan then turn out onto a plate.

Vegetable Stir-Fry

Serves 4

2 tbsp extra virgin olive oil

1 onion, chopped

1 garlic clove, sliced

1 small can water chestnuts (approx 225g/8oz)

2 tbsp wheat-free tamari sauce

¼ tsp sea salt

pepper

2 carrots, sliced

1 red pepper, deseeded and sliced

2 courgettes, sliced

½ medium-sized cauliflower, cut into florets

1 can chopped tomatoes (approx 450g/1lb)

1 large potato, chopped

25g/8oz/5 cups bean sprouts
rice, to serve, if desired

1 Heat a wok over medium heat and then add the oil. When
  hot, add the onion and garlic. Fry for around 5 minutes.
2 Add the water chestnuts and cook for a few minutes until
  tender, but still crisp.
3 Add the tamari sauce, seasoning and all the vegetables
  except the bean sprouts. Fry for 8–10 minutes before
  adding the bean sprouts. Cook for a further 2 minutes
  then serve hot with rice, if desired.

Salads

You'll be pleased to know that you can eat all the salads listed
in Chapter 4 (see page 48). In addition, you can also enjoy any
of the following salads, some of which include oats and rye.

Grated Vegetable and Raisin Munch

Serves 2

¼ celeriac, peeled and grated
2 medium carrots, grated
¼ small white cabbage, grated
1 spring onion, trimmed and sliced
75g/3oz/¾ cup raisins
3 tbsp wheat-free mayonnaise
2 sprigs garden mint, finely chopped
baked potatoes or lightly buttered rye bread, to serve

1 Place the grated vegetables and spring onion slices in a bowl, together with the raisins. Mix together to combine then stir in the mayonnaise.
2 Garnish with the chopped mint. Serve with baked potatoes or lightly buttered rye bread.

Stir-Fried Turkey, Orange and Basil Salad
Serves 4

finely grated zest and juice of 1 unwaxed orange
1 tsp wheat-free mustard
1 tbsp clear honey or agave syrup (see page 49)
450g/1lb turkey strips
2 tsp extra virgin olive oil
3 medium onions, thinly sliced
a handful of fresh basil, chopped
115g/4oz/½ cup cherry tomatoes, halved
2 oranges, peeled and segmented

1 In a bowl, mix together the orange zest and juice, mustard, honey or agave syrup and turkey strips. Leave to marinate for 30–40 minutes.
2 Heat the oil in a frying pan or wok over high heat for around 5 minutes until golden brown. Reduce the heat and add the onions, stirring. Cook until the onions are softened and golden brown. Add a little extra oil and cook the turkey strips, turning frequently to ensure they are thoroughly cooked.
3 Arrange the basil, tomatoes and orange segments on serving plates and distribute the turkey over the top. Drizzle with pan juices, if desired and serve immediately.

Iceberg Lettuce, Asparagus and Avocado Salad

Serves 4

Cornsalad is a variety of green leafy salad, available from health food shops, some supermarkets, as well as organic vegetable box delivery schemes

½ iceberg lettuce, shredded
1 small bunch cornsalad (also called lambs lettuce)
1 small bunch chives
1 small bunch garden mint
1 small bunch basil
1 large avocado, peeled, stoned and sliced
olive oil, for frying
200g/7oz tender asparagus, trimmed
wheat-free bread, oatcakes or 100% rye bread, to serve

Dressing:
2 tbsp olive oil
1 tbsp red wine or cider vinegar
2 garlic cloves, crushed
1 tsp clear honey
pinch of sea salt

1 Rinse and pat dry the lettuce and cornsalad.
2 Chop the chives and pick the leaves from mint and basil.
3 Place the lettuce and cornsalad in a bowl with the avocado and mix well.
4 Coat a frying pan with a little oil and cook the asparagus over a low heat until browned and slightly softened.
5 Place all of the ingredients for the dressing in a separate bowl. Whisk and blend together well.
6 Arrange the hot asparagus over the salad and pour the

dressing on top; toss together well. Serve with wheat-free bread, oatcakes or 100% rye bread.

Chickpea and Cashew Nut Salad
Serves 2

225g/8oz/1½ cups cooked chickpeas (or use ready-cooked canned chickpeas)
40g/1½oz/¼ cup cashew nut pieces
1 garlic clove, crushed
3 tbsp lemon juice
2 tbsp rapeseed oil
¼ tsp sea salt
1 Cos lettuce heart, shredded
a handful of fresh basil leaves, chopped
100% rye bread or wheat-free bread rolls, to serve

1 Drain the chickpeas into a bowl and mash until a coarse texture. Combine with the cashew nut pieces.
2 In a separate bowl, mix together the garlic, lemon juice, oil and salt; combine with the nut and chickpea mix.
3 Layer the lettuce over a serving plate and spoon the salad mix on top.
4 Garnish with the fresh basil and serve with 100% rye bread or wheat-free bread rolls.

Pasta, Haricot Bean and Tuna Salad

Serves 2

This is a high-protein, filling salad using wheat-free pasta. It is very suitable as a main dish.

400g/14oz/2 cups wheat-free pasta
255g/8oz canned kidney beans, drained
1 red onion, finely chopped
2 celery sticks, trimmed and finely chopped
50g/2oz/1½ cups walnuts, coarsely chopped
1 small can tuna in brine or oil (approx 200g/7oz)
3 tbsp extra virgin olive oil
3 tbsp cider vinegar
a pinch of sea salt
freshly ground black pepper
115g/4oz/2 cups shredded iceberg lettuce

1 Cook the pasta in boiling salted water according to the package directions. Rinse in cold water and drain into a bowl.
2 Add the kidney beans and combine with the pasta. Stir in the onion, celery and walnuts. Add the tuna and mix well
3 In a separate bowl or jug, combine the oil, vinegar and seasoning. Pour over the salad and toss together well.
4 Line a serving bowl with shredded lettuce and turn the mixture out into the centre; serve.

Wheat-Free Style Tabbouleh
Serves 2

175g/6oz/1 cup quinoa, rinsed
50g/2oz/1 cup fresh parsley, chopped
1 garlic clove, crushed
2 tbsp fresh mint, finely chopped
juice of 1 small lemon
700ml/25 fl oz/3 cups water
2 tbsp extra virgin olive oil
4 spring onions, trimmed and finely chopped
5 cherry tomatoes, quartered
a pinch of sea salt
freshly ground black pepper

1 Place the quinoa in a pan and cover with water, bring to the boil then reduce the heat and simmer for around 10–15 minutes until tender and all of the liquid is absorbed. Leave to cool. The grains will appear translucent and retain a slight bite when done.
2 Toss all the remaining ingredients together in a bowl and stir in the quinoa.
3 Leave to stand for 15 minutes to allow the flavours to infuse then serve.

Wild Rice and Icelandic Prawn Salad
Serves 4
Packets of wild rice usually come as a mix consisting of wild rice and long-grain rice. Icelandic prawns are my favourite because they are believed to come from waters that are less polluted.

115g/4oz/¾ cup wild rice
100g/3½oz/¼ cup button mushrooms, sliced
3 spring onions, trimmed and finely chopped
6 radishes, trimmed and sliced
130g/4½oz/1 cup cooked Icelandic prawns
wheat- or gluten-free French dressing, to serve

1 Cook the wild rice according to the directions on the package. Drain and rinse in cold water. Transfer to a serving bowl.
2 Add the mushrooms, spring onions, radishes and prawns. Mix well to combine and serve with the French dressing.

Tofu and Potato Salad
Serves 2

450g/1lb new potatoes, scrubbed
1 tbsp vegetable oil
1 tbsp wine vinegar or cider vinegar
1 small can (approx 200g/7oz) sweetcorn
1 small pot (approx 150g/5oz) plain yoghurt
a pinch of sea salt
freshly ground black pepper
115g/4oz/½ cup smoked tofu cubes
1 bunch watercress, trimmed
100% rye bread or rye crispbread, to serve, if desired

1 Place the potatoes in a large pan of salted water. Bring to the boil then reduce the heat and simmer until tender, about 15–20 minutes. Drain, dice into small chunks and place in a heatproof serving bowl.

2 Mix the oil and vinegar in a jug and pour over the hot potatoes. Mix well and leave to infuse

3 Drain the sweetcorn into a bowl and combine with the yoghurt and seasoning. Add smoked tofu to the potatoes, together with the sweetcorn-yoghurt dressing; mix well.

4 Spoon the salad onto a serving platter and garnish with the watercress. Serve with 100% rye bread or rye crispbread, if desired

Brown Rice Noodles with Broccoli, Carrots and Beetroot
Serves 2

200g/7oz packet brown rice noodles
150g/5oz/2 cups broccoli florets
115g/4oz/1 cup grated carrots
115g/4oz/1 cup grated beetroot
2 spring onions, trimmed and finely chopped
50ml/2 fl oz wheat-free tamari sauce

1 Boil the rice noodles in salted water according to the package directions. When almost cooked, add the broccoli and cook al dente. Drain and refresh in cold water. Transfer to a bowl.

2 Add the carrot, beetroot and spring onions. Stir in the tamari sauce; serve.

Quinoa, Apricots and Feta Salad
Serves 2

175g/6oz/1 cup quinoa, rinsed
4 ready-soaked unsulphured apricots
¼ tsp sea salt
100ml/3 1/2 fl oz/½ cup orange juice
200g/7oz/1⅓ cup feta cheese, cubed
3 tbsp olive oil

1 Place the quinoa in a saucepan and cover with salted water. Bring to the boil then reduce the heat and simmer for 10–15 minutes until tender and all the liquid has been absorbed.
2 Drain the quinoa and place in a bowl with the apricots and seasoning. Set aside.
3 Gently heat the orange juice in a saucepan and bring to the boil. Pour over the quinoa and leave to stand for about 10 minutes until absorbed.
4 Stir the quinoa mixture, ensuring all lumps are removed. Add the feta cheese and oil; mix well and serve.

Desserts
As with the main meal suggestions, there is a wide variety of wheat-free desserts, especially as many of your favourites do not usually contain any wheat products.

Baked Apples with Sultanas and Cinnamon
Serves 4

4 cooking apples, cored

grated zest and juice of 1 unwaxed orange
30g/1¼oz butter or margarine
1 tbsp clear honey or agave syrup (see page 49)
1 tsp cinnamon powder
bio-yoghurt or ice cream to serve, optional

1 Preheat the oven to 180°C/350°F/Gas 4.
2 Prick the skins of the apples at intervals and place in an ovenproof dish.
3 In a bowl, blend together the orange zest, juice, butter or margarine and honey or agave syrup. Pour the mixture carefully into the centre of the apples, sprinkle with cinnamon and cover the dish.
4 Bake for around 45 minutes in the centre of the oven or until the apples are cooked through. Serve with bio-yoghurt or ice cream, if desired.

Wheat-Free Chocolate Brownies
Makes 16

50g/2oz butter, softened at room temperature, plus extra
    to grease
150g/5oz/¾ cups wheat- or gluten-free flour
100g/3½oz/½ cup light brown sugar
1 tsp wheat-free baking powder
¼ tsp sea salt
1 tsp alcohol-free natural vanilla essence (available from health
    food shops)
2 medium eggs
100g/3½oz/½ cup apple purée
50g/2oz/½ cup cocoa powder

1   Preheat the oven to 180°C/350°F/Gas 4. Meanwhile, grease
    a cake tin measuring 8 x 20cm (3½ x 8in) square.
2   Place the flour, sugar, baking powder and salt in a bowl
    and mix thoroughly to combine.
3   In another bowl, place the butter, vanilla essence and eggs.
    Beat together for 1–2 minutes. Add the apple purée and beat
    to blend with the mixture then fold in the flour mixture.
4   Add the cocoa powder and blend again. Spoon the
    brownie mixture into the cake tin and bake in the oven for
    12–15 minutes. When cooked, divide into 16 squares and
    place on a wire rack to cool.

Oat and Sultana Flapjacks
Makes 16

115g/4oz butter, plus extra to grease
2 tbsp golden syrup
50g/2oz/¼ cup light brown sugar
225g/8oz/3¼ cups rolled oats
1 tbsp sultanas

1   Preheat the oven to 180ºC/350ºF/Gas 4 Meanwhile, place
    the butter, syrup and sugar in a saucepan and heat gently
    until melted, stirring occasionally. Remove from the heat
    and stir in the oats and sultanas to mix thoroughly.
2   Grease a 20cm (8in) square baking tin. Spoon in the oat
    mixture and flatten slightly. Bake in the centre of the oven
    for 20–25 minutes until golden brown.
3   Leave to cool slightly before dividing into 16 squares with
    a sharp knife. Store in an airtight container. They will keep
    in an airtight tin for five days.

Rice Pudding

Serves 2

This can be made with either wholegrain or white rice.

600ml/1 pint/3 cups skimmed milk
50g/2oz/¼ cup wholegrain or white shortgrain rice
25g/1oz/¼ cup dark Muscovado sugar
1 tsp alcohol free natural vanilla essence
½ tsp ground cinnamon
100g/3½oz/1 cup sultanas or raisins

1 Place the milk, rice, sugar, vanilla essence and cinnamon in a saucepan. Bring to the boil, stirring constantly.
2 Lower the heat and leave to simmer for 30–40 minutes until the grains are softened, adding the raisins for the final 10 minutes of cooking time.
3 Serve warm or leave to cool, refrigerate and serve cold later on.

Raspberry and Banana Sorbet

Serves 2

450g/1 lb/3 cups fresh raspberries, hulled
2 bananas, peeled and sliced
juice of 2 lemons
115g/4oz/1⅛ cups raw cane sugar

1 Blend the fruit in a liquidizer to form a purée.
2 In a bowl, mix the lemon juice with the sugar; blend with the fruit.
3 Pour into a freezerproof container and place in the freezer.

4 Remove after 1 hour and stir mixture to break up the ice crystals. Replace and leave to freeze fully.
5 Alternatively, you can churn in an electric ice-cream maker as per the manufacturer's instructions.
6 The sorbet will keep for two weeks.

Coconut, Date and Hazelnut Surprise
Serves 2

250ml/8 fl oz/1 cup water
125ml/4 fl oz/½ cup creamed coconut
175g/6oz/1 cup stoned dates, finely chopped
1 tsp alcohol free natural vanilla essence
75g/3oz/¾ cup chopped hazelnuts

1 Pour the water into a saucepan and bring to the boil? Stir in the creamed coconut and simmer.
2 Add the dates and stir them into the mixture. Cook over a very low heat, stirring occasionally until a smooth and creamy consistency.
3 Stir in the vanilla essence and the hazelnuts.
4 Transfer to a container and allow to cool. Chill in the refrigerator before serving.

Banana Fritters
Serves 2

115g/4oz/1½ cups wheat-free flour
a pinch of sea salt
1 egg, separated
1 tbsp extra virgin olive oil
150ml/5 fl oz/¾ cup milk
2 bananas
2 tbsp clear honey
1 tsp sweet spices (such as a mixture of nutmeg, cinnamon and
   vanilla) or allspice
extra virgin olive oil for frying
fresh or soya cream, to serve

1 Place the flour in a bowl and mix in the salt. Make a well
  in the centre. Add the egg yolk with a wooden spoon and
  beat in.
2 Gradually mix in the olive oil and then the milk in stages
  to achieve a smooth, creamy batter. Leave to stand for
  about 1½–2 hours in a cool position, then beat the egg
  white in a separate bowl and fold in to the mixture.
3 Chop the banana into 5cm (2in) slices.
4 Mix the honey with the sweet spices in a bowl and use to
  coat the banana slices.
5 Heat the oil on a medium heat for about 2 minutes in a
  shallow pan.
6 Dip in batter and deep-fry until golden brown, approximately 5 minutes. Serve with fresh or soya cream.

Honey and Nut Custard
Serves 2

2 medium eggs
125ml/4 fl oz honey or agave syrup (see page 49)
125ml/4 fl oz semi-skimmed milk
115g/4oz cashew nut butter
1 tbsp cornflour
a pinch of sea salt
butter or oil for greasing

1 Preheat the oven to 180°C/350°F/Gas 4. Place all the ingredients in a liquidiser and blend until smooth.
2 Spoon the mixture into a greased ovenproof dish (20cm x 20cm x 5cm/8"x 8"x 2")and bake for about 30 minutes until set. Serve hot or leave to cool and serve chilled.

Pecan Nut Yoghurt
Serves 2

250ml/9 fl oz plain bio-yoghurt
2 tbsp chopped pecan nuts
1 tbsp honey or agave syrup (see page 49)

Place the ingredients in a liquidiser and blend until smooth. Refrigerate for an hour or so to chill before serving.

Chocolate Mousse with Soya Cream

Serves 2

The use of soya cream in this recipe makes it a healthier alternative to ordinary dairy cream

115g/4oz good-quality dark chocolate

4 medium eggs, separated

1 tsp alcohol free natural vanilla essence

2 tbsp clear honey

150ml/¼ pint soya cream, to serve

1 Break the chocolate into pieces and warm in a heatproof bowl set over a pan of very hot water (or a double boiler) until completely melted.
2 Beat the egg whites in a bowl until stiff peaks form.
3 Stir the egg yolks into the chocolate, add the vanilla essence and mix in the honey and the beaten egg whites.
4 Spoon into individual glass dishes and refrigerate until set. Top with soya cream to serve.

Healthy wheat-free snacks

All the gluten-free snacks listed at the end of Chapter 4 (see page 60) can be also be eaten if you're on a wheat-free diet. In addition, you can have snacks that include 100% ryebread, rye crispbread (made from 100% rye flour), barley and barley malt.

6

Dairy intolerance

As far as dairy products are concerned, let me get straight to the point: milk is not the healthy food that the advertisements claim it to be. In fact, it is widely regarded by many authorities as being one of the most allergenic foods on the planet! Not surprisingly, I regularly encounter many clients with milk intolerance who also suffer a diverse range of health problems especially sinus congestion, skin conditions, asthma, ear infections and digestive complaints. Perhaps this is not surprising when you consider that cow's milk was meant for calves, not humans. What's more, humans are the only species on earth that feed on the milk of another species. Imagine a kitten feeding on elephant milk or a foal drinking milk from a giraffe? The composition would be wrong and health problems would be the end result. The same thing happens when babies are weaned onto cow's milk. This is known to increase the likelihood of a cow's milk allergy or intolerance, which is thought to affect as many as one in ten babies. Symptoms commonly experienced in babies include diarrhoea, persistent colic, eczema, urticaria, catarrh, sleeplessness and vomiting. This is consistent with the views of Dr Frank Oski, former director of the Department of Paediatrics at Johns Hopkins University School of Medicine and physician-in-chief of the Johns Hopkins Children's Center.

In his book, *Don't Drink Your Milk* (see page 302), Dr Oski states: 'The fact is: The drinking of cow milk has been linked with iron-deficiency anaemia in infants and children; it has been named as the cause of cramps and diarrhoea in much of the world's population, the cause of multiple forms of allergy as well.' In contrast, feeding an infant on breast milk reduces the chances of allergies and intolerances developing and also helps in normal development in all areas of the body including the brain, since it is known that breast-fed babies have an average of a four-point higher IQ. This can be further improved if the mother has a diet that is higher in healthy fats, especially omega 3 essential fatty acids (these are derived from fish oils and some nuts and seeds – for example, flaxseeds or linseeds).

The nutritious milk fallacy

Despite all the hype about milk being such a nutritious food for humans, the reality turns out to be somewhat different. For instance, milk is not a good source of magnesium, manganese and selenium whereas in comparison fruits and vegetables are a much better source of these minerals. Milk is certainly high in calcium, containing about 1,200mg in just over 1 litre (1¾ pints). The same amount of human milk contains about 300mg calcium. However, a human infant will absorb much more of the calcium from breast milk compared to the same amount of cow's milk. This is because the cow's milk contains a high amount of phosphorous that inhibits calcium absorption. Also, cow's milk is low in magnesium in relation to calcium. Humans need magnesium to absorb calcium efficiently. Needless to say, the magnesium:calcium ratio is much better in breast milk and helps with calcium uptake by the infant (also the case with adults). This means the high amount of calcium in cow's milk cannot be used. Sometimes this results in calcium being left in soft tissues and joints, a condition known as 'calcium dumping syndrome' or it can build up in the form of kidney stones.

Bearing the above in mind, you may not be too surprised to learn that cow's milk has been linked with a higher incidence of osteoporosis – the very condition it is supposed to help! Apart from the aforementioned imbalance between calcium and magnesium, it is known that cow's milk contains proteins that produce acid end products in the body. In response to this the body ends up robbing calcium from the bones to neutralise acids. The end result is weakened bones that are more prone to osteoporosis!

Milk and mucous

Are you one of those people who wakes up feeling congested in the morning? Do you experience sinus pains, perhaps resulting in sinus headaches? Maybe you suffer from frequent head colds? If so, it could be that your diet contains too many mucous-forming foods or you may have an intolerance that can lead to an increase in mucous production in the body. Even if you're not intolerant to milk, it's worth remembering that it is probably the most mucous-forming food of all. In fact, I've lost count of the number of people I've encountered that suffer from mucous congestion of one sort or another. Invariably, when they omit dairy foods from their diet, they experience great relief from their symptoms. I remember one lady who had a persistent cough that just wouldn't go away. She was most embarrassed by this because she worked in a small office and she felt that her constant coughing was disturbing her colleagues. She had already eliminated gluten from her diet and that had improved the situation. However, she was still left with the annoying cough. I advised her to reduce the amount of mucous-forming foods in her diet, especially dairy products. She did as I suggested and within a week or so her cough had almost entirely disappeared.

Health conditions commonly associated with intolerance to dairy products

The components in milk that are most likely to cause an allergy or intolerance include lactose (milk sugar), casein (a milk protein) and lactalbumin (milk protein). As stated earlier, sometimes intolerance to lactose is the result of a lack of lactase, which is an enzyme in the body that is needed to break it down. In such cases it's still advisable to avoid milk and its products; however, some people may overcome the problem if they take a supplement of the enzyme lactase, usually in the form of tablets.

If you suspect that you may have a problem with digesting milk and milk products, I would advise you to consult your doctor to establish whether you might be lactase deficient. Here is a list of symptoms that might indicate that you are intolerant to dairy products. Remember these include milk and milk products from cow's, goat's, ewe's and buffalo milk; also milk, cheese, yoghurt and whey.

- Irritable Bowel Syndrome (IBS)
- Constipation
- Bloating
- Nausea
- Flatulence

- Indigestion
- Acid reflux
- Abdominal pain
- Skin conditions – hives, nettle rash, eczema
- Chronic runny nose
- Nasal congestion
- Sinus congestion and sinus pain
- Recurring bronchitis
- Frequent colds
- Asthma
- Ear infections
- Coughing
- Irritability
- Colic in infants
- May interfere with normal physical development in some infants and children
- Weight regulation problems

As with the other food intolerances I've covered so far in this book, the above list is not exhaustive. If you suspect that you might have dairy intolerance then it's important that you get tested, or omit dairy foods 100% from your diet for a three-day trial then note the result.

Foods to avoid on a dairy-free diet

- Milk
- Buttermilk
- Cheese
- Yoghurt
- Whey and whey solids
- Milk solids
- Skimmed milk
- Any substance ending in 'caseinate' such as calcium or sodium caseinate, which is used in the manufacture of some baked and fried foods, ice creams and processed meats.
- Cream
- Butter
- Lactose
- Lactalbumin
- Lactoglobulin
- Curds

103

Hidden milk products

In addition to the foregoing list, you'll need to look out for the following foods that may contain milk in its variety of forms:

- Bakery products such as bread, biscuits, muffins, crackers, etc.
- Sauces
- Gravy powder
- Beverages such as hot drinks (for example night-time drinks made from powder)

- Fondues
- Cereals
- Margarine (some brands may contain milk solids)
- Confectionery
- Ready-meals
- Sausages
- Canned meats

Once you become familiar with the ingredients to look out for, you'll find that sticking to a dairy-free diet is not as difficult as it might at first appear. Here is a typical ingredients list that you may encounter in a product such as a chocolate spread. The milk product is hidden among the other ingredients so it is worthwhile checking closely.

> Ingredients: Sugar, soya oil, peanuts (13%), fat-reduced cocoa powder, skimmed milk powder (7.0%), soy lecithin (emulsifier), flavouring.

Remember, though: many products make it easy for you by stating 'dairy-free' on the can, bottle or package. If in any doubt, scrutinise the ingredients list.

Dairy-free substitutes

Fortunately, as with gluten- and wheat-free foods, a growing number of dairy-free alternatives are available. These include:

- Soya milk
- Rice milk
- Almond milk
- Dairy-free cheese
- Dairy-free spreads, including margarines

- Dairy-free ice cream
- Soya yoghurt
- Soya cream
- Soya desserts

PLEASE NOTE

If you've glanced over the preceding gluten- and wheat-free recipes in this book, you'll have noticed that I have included dairy ingredients in some of the dishes. In some ways this was a difficult decision for me to make, given my awareness of the disadvantages associated with dairy products. Nevertheless, I have included them because I see no value in being too purist regarding their inclusion. Besides, I'm also aware that an individual who is trying to avoid, let's say wheat, will have enough to think about without worrying too much about trying to omit dairy products as well. However, I'm a great believer in giving people the information they require so that they can make their own informed choices. In this regard, you do have the option of substituting milk products with suitable dairy-free alternatives if you prefer to do so. Of course, the following recipes are all entirely free from dairy products, however:

Dairy-free recipes

There are up to 10 million people in the UK alone who would benefit from following a milk or lactose-free diet. But you don't have to forego any of your favourite dishes.

Breakfast
Although milk products are frequently used in many breakfast dishes, as you'll see from the recipes that follow, there are numerous dairy-free alternatives which means you can enjoy a different one every day.

Nut and Raisin Soya Yoghurt
Serves 2
This is a simple and delicious alternative to ordinary yoghurt. It is prepared the night before and refrigerated.

250ml/9 fl oz plain soya yoghurt
I tbsp clear honey or agave syrup (see page 49)
3 tbsp raisins
50g/2oz/½ cup chopped hazelnuts

1 Pour the yoghurt into a bowl and add the honey or syrup.
2 Stir in the raisins and hazelnuts and refrigerate overnight. In the morning, give the mixture a stir and serve.

Potato Pancakes
Makes 6
The pancakes can be served with grilled tomatoes or pile mounds of potato on toast.

4 medium potatoes, grated
I onion, thinly sliced
I tbsp wholemeal or white flour
I tbsp wholemeal breadcrumbs
I tbsp soya cream cheese
I egg, lightly beaten
I tsp sea salt
freshly ground black pepper
I tbsp extra virgin olive oil

1 In a large bowl, mix together the grated potatoes and the sliced onion.
2 Add the flour, breadcrumbs, soya cream cheese, egg and seasoning. Mix thoroughly to combine.
3 Heat the oil in a frying pan and spread the pancake mixture evenly on top using a spatula. Fry until brown on both sides, about 2 minutes each.

Spicy Dried Fruit and Soya Yoghurt Delight
Serves 2

3 tbsp mixed vine fruit, presoaked in water overnight
250ml/9 fl oz plain soya yoghurt
I tsp ground mixed spice

Divide the fruit into 2 breakfast bowls and layer with the soya yoghurt. Sprinkle with ground mixed spice and serve.

Granola

Serves 2–3

A delicious crunchy breakfast cereal: serve with soya yoghurt or any dairy-free milk.

575g/1¼lb/4 cups rolled oats

115g/4oz/1 cup sultanas

75g/3oz/1 cup desiccated coconut

150g/5oz/1 cup sunflower seeds

150g/5oz/1 cup cashew-nut pieces

75g/3oz/½ cup sesame seeds

115g/4oz/1 cup wheatgerm

½ tsp sea salt

4 tbsp vegetable oil, plus extra to grease

125ml/4 fl oz clear honey

1 Preheat the oven to 160°C/325°F/Gas 3. Combine all the dry ingredients together in a large, heatproof bowl.

2 In a small saucepan, gently heat the vegetable oil and add the honey, stirring well. Pour over the dry ingredients and mix in with your fingertips to achieve a crumbly consistency.

3 Lightly grease a baking sheet or tray and spread the mixture evenly over the surface. Heat in the oven for about 15 minutes until lightly browned, using a spatula to turn the mixture halfway through cooking time.

4 When cooled, store in an airtight container, where it will keep for approximately two weeks.

Dairy-Free Scrambled Eggs
Serves 1

2 eggs
1½ tbsp soya milk (or other milk substitute if preferred)
pinch of sea salt
freshly ground black pepper
1 tbsp dairy-free margarine
wholemeal or white bread toast, to serve

1 Beat the eggs in a bowl with the milk and season.
2 Melt the margarine in a saucepan over a low heat. Pour in the eggs and continue to gently heat, stirring with a wooden spoon, until the eggs are scrambled to your liking. Serve with wholemeal or white bread toast.

Almond Butter and Honey Toastie
Serves 1
This breakfast option is both quick to prepare and nutritious. If wholemeal bread is used, this will provide long-term energy as the sugars are released more slowly.

2 slices wholemeal or white bread
1 tbsp dairy-free margarine
1 tsp honey
40g/1½oz almond butter

1 Coat one side of each bread slice with margarine.
2 Blend the honey with the almond butter and spread over the other side of the bread slices.

3 Form into a sandwich and toast in a sandwich maker for about 5 minutes. Serve hot.

Grilled Banana and Soya Cream
Serves 1

1 or 2 medium bananas, peeled and halved lengthways
50ml/2 fl oz soya cream
¼ tsp ground cinnamon
1 tbsp chopped hazelnuts, optional

1 Preheat the grill to medium. Place the banana(s) underneath and grill until slightly browned, turning once. Transfer to a breakfast bowl.
2 Spoon soya cream on top and sprinkle with cinnamon and hazelnuts, if desired. Serve while still warm.

Banana and Strawberry Soya Cream Smoothie
Serves 1
This is a dairy-free version of a thick and creamy smoothie, substituting soya cream for whole milk.

1 medium or large banana, peeled and sliced
225ml/8 fl oz/1 cup soya or almond milk
50ml/2 fl oz/¼ cup soya cream
175g/6oz/1 cup strawberries, hulled
1 tsp clear honey or agave syrup (see page 49)

1 Place all the ingredients except the honey in a blender or smoothie maker. Blend until creamy smooth.

2 Drizzle with honey or agave syrup and blend again. Serve immediately.

Main meals

The good news is that there are many delicious recipes for main meals that do not rely on dairy products. And the even better news is that those that do, can be easily adapted by substituting with a dairy-free alternative.

Vegetable Soya Soup

Serves 2

3 tbsp olive oil
I onion, finely diced
I small can (approx 200g/7oz) chopped tomatoes
2 courgettes, sliced
I red pepper, deseeded and finely chopped
¼ tsp sea salt
I tbsp chopped fresh herbs or I tsp mixed dried herbs
4 tbsp soya flour
2 tbsp wholemeal flour
900ml/1½ pints/4½ cups dairy-free vegetable stock
I tbsp tamari sauce
wholemeal or white bread, to serve

1 Gently heat the olive oil in a large frying pan. Add the onion and sauté until golden then stir in the chopped tomatoes, courgettes, pepper, sea salt and herbs.
2 When well cooked, stir in the soya and wholemeal flour and cook for a few minutes more.
3 Add the stock a little at a time, stirring to prevent the

formation of lumps. When all the stock is added, bring to the boil and add the tamari sauce. Reduce the heat and simmer for 12–15 minutes. Serve with wholemeal or white bread

Vegetable Kebabs
Serves 2

2 large aubergines, diced into 2.5cm/1in cubes
sea salt
225g/8oz small onions or shallots, peeled
2 red or yellow peppers, deseeded and cut into 2.5cm/1in squares
5 tomatoes, halved
225g/8oz button mushrooms, wiped
2 courgettes, sliced
1 tbsp extra virgin olive oil (or other vegetable oil)
freshly ground black pepper
a salad of spinach, red chard, rocket and red cos lettuce to serve

1 Rinse the aubergines in a colander and sprinkle lightly with sea salt. Leave to drain for 15–20 minutes, then rinse in cold water.
2 Par-boil the aubergine with the onions or shallots in a saucepan of water for about 10 minutes, drain.
3 Preheat the grill to medium-high. Meanwhile, skewer all the vegetables alternately together and brush lightly with the oil using a pastry brush.
4 Sprinkle with seasoning and grill, basting with oil every so often and turning so they are cooked evenly. When ready, they should be a light brown colour and tender.
5 Serve with the salad a healthy dressing such as French dressing.

Nutty Potato Burgers

Serves 2

Serve with your favourite cooked vegetables or a salad of grated carrot, iceberg lettuce and finely chopped red onions.

225g/8oz potatoes, peeled

2 tbsp extra virgin olive oil, plus extra for grilling

1 medium red onion, sliced

115g/4oz mushrooms, wiped and sliced

2 tbsp dairy-free margarine

a pinch of sea salt

freshly ground black pepper

115g/4oz chopped nuts such as hazelnuts or walnuts

1 tbsp finely chopped parsley

1 Place the potatoes in a large saucepan and cover with boiling, salted water. Bring to the boil and then simmer for 15–20 minutes until cooked.

2 Meanwhile, heat the oil in a frying pan and sauté the onion and mushrooms until golden. Set aside.

3 When cooked, mash the potatoes in the saucepan with the margarine and season. Stir in the cooked onion, mushrooms, chopped nuts and parsley.

4 Preheat the grill to medium. Meanwhile, shape the potato mixture into six burger shapes. Brush lightly with oil and grill for about 10 minutes, turning at the half way stage, until golden brown.

5 Serve with the vegetables or a lightly-dressed salad.

Lentil and Sweet Potato Pie
Serves 2

375g/12oz/2¼ cups puy lentils, soaked
225g/8oz sweet potatoes, peeled and cut into chunks
20g/¾oz dairy-free margarine
a pinch of sea salt
freshly ground black pepper
1 tbsp olive oil for frying
   Plus 1 tbsp extra for greasing
1 onion, chopped
1 small can (approx 200g/7oz) chopped tomatoes
50ml/2 fl oz/¼ cup soya or other dairy-free milk
vegetables, to serve

1 Preheat the oven to 190°C/375°F/Gas 5. Meanwhile, cook the lentils in a saucepan of water for 20 minutes until tender, drain and set aside.
2 Place the sweet potatoes in a large saucepan and add enough boiled salted water to cover. Bring to the boil then reduce the heat and simmer until cooked, about 15–20 minutes. Drain, return to the pan and mash with the margarine and soya or dairy-free milk; season.
3 Heat the oil in a frying pan and sauté the onion until softened. Stir in the chopped tomatoes and simmer gently for a few more minutes.
4 Lightly grease a casserole dish and layer the lentils in the base then add the onion and tomatoes. Spread mashed sweet potato over the top. Bake for 25–30 minutes until golden brown on top.
Serve with your favourite lightly cooked vegetables such as carrots, courgettes and cauliflower.

'Eggy' Spinach Pie

Serves 2

Ideally served with cooked vegetables such as carrots, red cabbage, peas or broccoli, or if eating cold, with a salad

2 tbsp vegetable oil, plus extra to grease
3 medium onions, chopped
4 eggs
200ml/7 fl oz/1 cup soya milk
a pinch of sea salt
freshly ground black pepper
3 tbsp chopped basil
800g/1¾lb spinach, finely chopped
40g/1½oz/¼ cup garden peas
115g/4oz dairy-free Cheddar, grated

1 Preheat the oven to 190°C/375°F/Gas 5. Meanwhile, heat the vegetable oil in a frying pan and gently fry the onions until softened. Set aside.
2 Beat the eggs in a bowl with the soya milk; season and stir in the chopped basil.
3 In another bowl, combine the spinach, onion and peas; transfer to an oiled pie dish. Pour the egg mixture over the top and top with grated cheese.
4 Bake for about 30 minutes until the vegetables are tender and the top browned.

Fried Fish and Homemade Chips

Serves 4

Good with peas, sweetcorn or grilled tomatoes.

4 fillets of white fish (cod, hake or haddock)
40g/1½oz/¼ cup wholemeal or white flour
freshly ground black pepper
5 medium potatoes, scrubbed, unpeeled and cut into chunky chips
extra virgin olive oil (or other oil of your choice)
1 tsp paprika
½ tsp sea salt

1 Preheat the oven to 200°C/400°F/Gas 6. Lightly coat the fish with flour on both sides and sprinkle with pepper.

2 Parboil the potato chips in boiling, salted water for 2–3 minutes. Drain and leave to cool. Spread out evenly on a non-stick baking sheet and drizzle with oil.

3 Dust with paprika and sea salt. Bake for 25–30 minutes, turning occasionally, until golden brown.

4 Meanwhile, lightly coat a frying pan with oil, heat through and gently cook the fish, turning once with a fish slice, until it is cooked through and slightly browned for about 5 minutes on each side or until it flakes. Transfer to a heatproof dish, cover and keep warm while you make the chips.

5 Serve the fish and chips with vegetables of your choice.

Spicy Cod with Beans and Rice

Serves 4

1 tbsp extra virgin olive oil

116

700g/1½lb cod fillet, skinned, cut into pieces and large bones
  removed
1 large can (approx 450g/1lb) chopped tomatoes
1 tbsp tomato paste
250g/9oz canned chopped French beans, drained
½ tsp chilli powder
½ tsp clear honey
wholegrain rice, to serve

1 Heat the oil in a large frying pan and fry the cod for 4–5
  minutes on each side until cooked through. Remove with
  a fish slice and keep warm.
2 Add the remaining ingredients apart from the rice to the
  pan and mix to combine thoroughly. Top with the fish,
  cover with a lid and simmer for 5–6 minutes or until the
  fish is tender.
3 Serve on a bed of cooked wholegrain rice with other
  cooked vegetables such as steamed broccoli, if desired.

Dairy-Free Macaroni Cheese with Turkey
Serves 4

1 medium onion
150ml/¼ pint/¾ cup vegetable stock
25g/1oz dairy-free margarine
25g/1oz/⅓ cup plain wholemeal or white flour
225ml/8 fl oz/1¼ cups soya milk
½ tsp sea salt
freshly ground black pepper
50g/2oz dairy-free Cheddar
225g/8oz wholemeal or white macaroni

4 ready-cooked turkey rashers (available from supermarkets)
4 tomatoes, sliced
3 tbsp fresh chopped basil
I tbsp dairy-free Parmesan, grated

1 Place the onion and stock in a large frying pan and bring to the boil, stirring occasionally. Reduce the heat and simmer for about 5 minutes until the onion is tender and the stock has completely reduced.
2 Mix together the margarine, flour, milk and seasoning until a smooth texture is achieved. Pour into a saucepan and gently heat, stirring, until the mixture thickens. Remove from the heat and add the Cheddar cheese and onion-stock mixture.
3 Cook the macaroni in a pan of boiling salted water according to the directions on the package. When cooked, drain and stir the sauce into the pan. Transfer to an ovenproof casserole.
4 Preheat the grill to high. Meanwhile, top the macaroni cheese with turkey rashers and sliced tomatoes. Sprinkle with basil and Parmesan cheese. Grill until the top is slightly browned and serve hot.

'Herby' Fried Rice
Serves 2

2 tbsp vegetable oil
I onion, sliced
400g/14oz/2 cups cooked brown rice
I tsp turmeric
I tsp tamari sauce

freshly ground black pepper

3 tbsp fresh chopped mixed herbs such as chives or basil

I small can (approx 200g/7oz) sweetcorn

2 courgettes, sliced

I large can (approx 450g/1lb) natural baked beans

1 Heat a little of the oil in a frying pan and gently fry the onion until tender. Remove from the pan and keep warm.

2 Mix together the rice, turmeric, tamari sauce, black pepper, herbs, sweetcorn and courgettes in a bowl. Add the remaining oil to the pan and fry the mixture over low to medium heat for 5–10 minutes until heated through and the vegetables are tender.

3 Transfer the rice mixture to a serving dish and keep warm.

4 Empty the canned beans into a saucepan and gently heat for 5 minutes. Serve with the rice.

Risotto
Serves 2

2 tbsp vegetable oil

I onion, chopped

I red pepper, deseeded and sliced

I yellow pepper, deseeded and sliced

I garlic clove, crushed

200g/7oz/1 cup brown or white rice

I tbsp yeast extract

550ml/18 fl oz/2¾ cups dairy-free vegetable stock, kept hot in a saucepan

2 tbsp fresh mixed herbs such as basil, thyme and chives

¼ tsp sea salt

freshly ground black pepper
115g/4oz dairy-free Cheddar, grated

1 Heat the oil in a frying pan and gently fry the onion, sliced peppers and garlic. When softened, add the rice and cook for around 5–6 minutes, stirring.
2 Dissolve the yeast extract into the stock and add the herbs and seasoning. Pour half the stock over the rice.
3 Continue to cook over low heat, gradually adding more stock as it is reduced. After about 15 minutes, when the rice is tender, stir in half the grated cheese and when melted, remove from the heat. Sprinkle with the remaining cheese and serve.

Salads
Any of the salads from the previous chapters are suitable for a dairy-free diet, provided you substitute dairy-free ingredients, where necessary. Here are some more ideas for salads that include dairy-free ingredients, where appropriate:

Green salads
There's no need for green salads to be dull with so many different combinations and an equally wide variety of accompanying ingredients that you can use. Choose from all types of lettuce, endive, chicory, spinach (including baby leaf), corn salad (a type of green, leafy salad plant), watercress, cabbage, cress, etc. You can also add interesting flavours with sprouted seeds such as alfalfa, radish sprouts and fenugreek. Here is one example:

Green Leaf and Root Vegetable Salad
Serves 2
Good with a baked potato filled with grated dairy-free cheese
or tuna.

175g/6oz/3 cups shredded iceberg lettuce
50g/2oz/2 cups alfalfa sprouts
1 medium red onion, finely chopped
50g/2oz/1 cup baby spinach
50g/2oz/1 cup corn salad, chopped
1 carrot, grated
1 beetroot, grated
75g/3oz/½ cup sunflower seeds
25g/1oz cup finely chopped garden mint
4 tbsp dairy-free salad dressing

1 Arrange the iceberg lettuce, alfalfa sprouts, spinach, corn
  salad and onion in a bowl and mix with your favourite
  dairy-free salad dressing such as French dressing.
2 Divide between plates and spread grated carrots and
  beetroot over the top.
3 Sprinkle with sunflower seeds and chopped mint, then
  drizzle a little extra dressing on top. Serve immediately.

Greek Tofu Salad
Serves 1
This is a good alternative to conventional Greek salad with
tofu as a substitute for feta cheese.

2 beef tomatoes, sliced
1 large green pepper, deseeded and sliced

1 onion, sliced
50g/2oz stoned black or green olives
115g/4oz/½ cup smoked or plain tofu chunks
oil and vinegar dressing (1 part vinegar to 2 parts oil, salt, pepper to
    serve

In a salad bowl, layer slices of tomatoes, green pepper and onion. Add the olives and tofu chunks. Serve drizzled with the oil and vinegar dressing.

Apple, Sultana and Walnut Salad
Serves 2
Good with corn chips or wholemeal bread.

4 eating apples, cored and sliced
juice of one lemon
3 sticks of celery, trimmed and chopped
3 tbsp sultanas
100g/3½oz/1cup walnut pieces
3 tbsp dairy-free mayonnaise or plain soya yoghurt

1. Place the apples in a bowl and soak in the lemon juice for 10 minutes.
2. Add the celery, sultanas and walnut pieces; mix well
3. Serve with mayonnaise or plain soya yoghurt.

Spicy Stuffed Eggs
Serves 2

4 eggs, hard-boiled and sliced in half lengthways
30g/1¼oz dairy-free margarine
¼ tsp sea salt
½ tsp chilli powder
juice of ½ lemon
1 tbsp grated dairy-free cheese
50g/2oz black or green stoned olives, finely chopped
1 tbsp pimentos
1 tsp chopped fresh parsley
wholemeal bread or white toasted bread, thinly spread with dairy-
    free margarine, to serve

1 Remove the yolks from the eggs. Mix together in a bowl
  with the margarine, seasoning, chilli powder, lemon juice,
  grated cheese and olives.
2 Fill the egg whites with the mixture and decorate with
  pimentos and parsley. Serve with wholemeal or white
  toasted bread.

Artichoke and Red Potato Salad
Serves 2

400g/14oz red potatoes
3 tbsp extra virgin olive oil
75g/3oz/½ cup walnuts, chopped
1 large can (approx 450g/1lb) artichoke hearts
175g/6oz/3 cups chopped iceberg lettuce leaves
2 courgettes, sliced

1 tbsp finely chopped fresh garden mint
juice of 1 lemon
a pinch of sea salt
freshly ground black pepper

1 Place the potatoes in a saucepan and cover with boiling, salted water. Bring to the boil, then reduce the heat and simmer until tender. Drain, quarter, return to the pan and coat with 1 tbsp oil.
2 Add the walnuts and mix well.
3 Drain the artichoke hearts. Arrange the lettuce with the potatoes and walnuts on a platter. Top with courgettes and artichoke hearts. Sprinkle over the chopped mint.
4 Mix the remaining olive oil, lemon juice and seasoning in a bowl. Drizzle over the salad and serve.

Avocado, Mushroom and Wild Rice Salad
Serves 2

1 garlic clove, crushed
juice of 2 small lemons
3 tbsp extra virgin olive oil
2 tsp mustard
375g/12oz/3 cups button mushrooms, thinly sliced
175g/6oz/3 cups alfalfa (or alfalfa and fenugreek sprouts)
1 medium carrot, grated
3 medium ripe avocados, peeled and sliced lengthways, then
    sprinkled with lemon juice to prevent browning
450g/1lb/3 cups cooked wild rice

1 In a bowl, whisk together the garlic, lemon juice, oil and mustard to make a dressing.
2 Stir in the mushrooms and leave to marinate for 30 minutes.
3 Arrange a bed of the alfalfa sprouts and grated carrot on each plate and layer avocado slices on top. Spoon the mushroom mixture over the avocado salad and serve with the wild rice.

Red Cabbage and Apple Salad
Serves 2

2 eating apples, cored
juice of I lemon
225g/8oz/3 cups shredded red cabbage
2 spring onions, finely chopped
I tsp cumin seeds
I tbsp extra virgin olive oil
a pinch of sea salt
freshly ground black pepper
2 tbsp almonds, chopped
I tbsp hazelnuts, chopped
I tbsp chopped chives
rye crispbread or rye bread, to serve

1 Grate the apples and coat with lemon juice to prevent browning.
2 In a bowl, mix together the apples, shredded cabbage and the spring onions. Sprinkle with cumin seeds and drizzle with oil; season.
3 Sprinkle with almonds and hazelnuts then garnish with chives. Serve with rye crispbread or rye bread.

Crab Salad
Serves 4

225ml/8 fl oz/1⅓ cups dairy-free mayonnaise
110ml/4 fl oz/½ cup soya cream
1 tsp chilli powder
1 onion, chopped
1 iceberg lettuce
450g/1lb/4 cups crabmeat, cooked
1 yellow or red pepper, deseeded and sliced
2 tbsp stoned black or green olives
3 tbsp chopped fresh chives
juice of ½ lemon

1 To make the dressing, blend the mayonnaise, soya cream and chilli powder together in a bowl until smooth.
2 Arrange the remaining ingredients in a serving bowl, sprinkle with chives and lemon juice and serve with the dressing.

Pasta and Turkey Salad
Serves 2

3 spring onions, trimmed and chopped
10 stoned black olives, halved
1 red or yellow pepper, deseeded and chopped
3 slices wholewheat bread
225g/8oz/2 cups cooked wholewheat pasta
2 tbsp extra virgin olive oil, plus extra for frying
225g/8oz/1½ cups turkey pieces
2 tbsp cider vinegar

1 tbsp tamari sauce
1 tsp dried basil
1 garlic clove, crushed

1 In a serving bowl, mix together the spring onions, olives and pepper; set aside.
2 Toast the bread and cut into small squares. Add the bread and pasta to the serving bowl.
3 Heat the olive oil in a frying pan and fry the turkey pieces for a few minutes until slightly brown and thoroughly cooked. Add to the salad mixture; stir to combine.
4 In another bowl, whisk together 2 tbsp extra virgin olive oil, vinegar, tamari, basil and garlic; mix well. Pour over the salad and toss before serving.

Dairy-Free desserts

Although dairy produce tends to figure quite prominently in desserts, there is always the option of using a dairy-free alternative – for example, almond milk, or soya cream. Coconut cream is also another option for some recipes. Be careful to purchase the brands containing no milk products, however.

Bread and 'Butter' Pudding
Serves 2
This version of the favourite pudding uses dairy-free margarine instead of butter.

50g/2oz dairy-free margarine, plus extra to grease
6 slices wholewheat bread
225g/8oz/2 cups sultanas or raisins
grated zest of 1 unwaxed lemon

1 tsp ground mixed spice

2 medium eggs

450ml/¾ pint/2¼ cups soya milk

100ml/3½ fl oz/1 cup soya cream

2 tbsp raw Muscovado sugar

1 Butter the bread on both sides and arrange in layers sprinkled with sultanas or raisins and lemon zest in a greased ovenproof dish. Sprinkle with the sweet spices.

2 In a bowl, beat the eggs with the soya milk, soya cream and sugar until the sugar has completely dissolved. Pour over the bread and stand for 45–50 minutes.

3 Preheat the oven to 150°C/300°F/Gas 2. Bake the pudding for 1 hour.

Hazelnut Flapjacks

Makes 12

225g/8oz dairy-free margarine, plus extra to grease

225g/8oz raw Muscovado sugar

¼ tsp sea salt

375g/12oz/2⅛ cups rolled oats

1 tbsp molasses

115g/4oz/1 cup chopped hazelnuts

1 Preheat the oven to 180°C/350°F/Gas 4. Meanwhile, gently heat the margarine in a frying pan and stir in the sugar and salt; set aside.

2 Mix together the oats, molasses and hazelnuts in a mixing bowl. Stir in the contents of the frying pan and mix well to combine.

3 Spoon the mixture onto a greased baking tray and spread out evenly with a palette knife.

4 Bake in the centre of the oven for about 20 minutes or until golden brown. Cool, then cut into 12 rectangles.

Dairy-Free Cream

Serves 4

This is a great alternative to ordinary cream. Use instead of ordinary cream with fruit puddings, rice puddings, etc.

225g/8oz firm silken tofu
4 tbsp clear honey or agave syrup (see page 49)
2 tbsp soya milk
I tsp vanilla extract

Place all the ingredients in a blender and blend for a few minutes until smooth. Transfer to a plastic container and chill for an hour or longer, if possible. This should keep for 2–3 days in the refrigerator.

Almond Milk Strawberry and Banana Smoothie

Serves 2

75g/3oz/½ cup chopped strawberries
200ml/7 fl oz/I cup almond milk
I tsp clear honey or agave syrup (see page 49)

Place all the ingredients in a blender or smoothie maker. Blend for a few minutes until smooth and serve in tall glasses.

Chilled Coconut and Carob Cookies
Makes 6–8
This recipe includes carob, which has a chocolate-like flavour.

50g/2oz dairy-free margarine, plus extra to grease
30g/11/4oz/¼ cup raw Muscovado sugar
150g/5oz/1 cup wholewheat flour
½ tsp baking powder
a pinch of salt
60ml/2½ fl oz/⅓ cup soya or almond milk
2 tbsp carob flour
50g/2oz/¾ cup desiccated coconut

1 Cream the margarine and sugar together in a mixing bowl
  until light and fluffy.
2 In another bowl, mix together the flour, baking powder
  and salt. Stir in the milk and then the carob flour followed
  by the coconut; mix thoroughly. Now add the margarine
  and sugar mixture.
3 Knead into a dough and then shape into a large sausage
  shape. Cover with foil and chill in the refrigerator for an hour.
4 When thoroughly chilled, remove the foil and slice into
  5cm/2in rounds. Preheat the oven to 160°C/325°F/Gas 3.
  Meanwhile, grease a baking tray and place the rounds on top.
  Bake for 10–12 minutes, remove from the oven and leave for
  a couple of minutes, then place in a wire rack to cool.

Almond Butter Oaties
Serves 4–6

50g/2oz margarine, plus extra to grease
50g/2oz almond nut butter
50g/2oz/½ cup rolled oats
65g/21/2oz/½ cup wholewheat or white flour
¼ tsp baking powder
3 tbsp water
50g/2oz/½ cup raw Muscovado sugar
a pinch of sea salt

1 Place the margarine and almond butter in a mixing bowl and beat together well.
2 Add the oats, flour, baking powder and water; mix together thoroughly.
3 Preheat the oven to 190°C/375°F/Gas 5. Meanwhile, lightly grease a baking tray and level the mixture to about 2.5cm/1in deep.
4 Bake for about 20 minutes until set. Remove from the oven, allow to cool for a couple of minutes, then place on a wire rack. Cut into rectangular bars.

Banana and Date Cake
Serves 6–8

225g/8oz/2 cups wholewheat or white flour
2 tsp baking powder
8 large dates, pitted and soaked in water for 1 hour
110ml/4 fl oz/½ cup water
225ml/8 fl oz/1 cup rice milk
110ml/4 fl oz/½ cup sunflower or safflower oil
2 ripe bananas, mashed
1 tbsp cider vinegar
1 tbsp margarine for greasing

1 Preheat the oven to 180°C/350°F/Gas 4. Meanwhile, in a bowl mix together the flour and baking powder.
2 In a blender, blend the dates with the water until a thick, creamy consistency is produced.
3 Fold the date mixture into the flour and add the rice milk, oil and bananas; mix well.
4 Finally, stir in the vinegar and pour the mixture into a greased 8inch/20cm round cake tin.
5 Bake in the centre of the oven for about 45 minutes. Test the cake with a skewer. If mixture sticks to it, return to the oven for a few more minutes.
6 Turn out onto a wire rack and leave to cool, then cut into slices.

Banana and Nut Ice Lollies
Makes 9

3 bananas
18g/2/3oz/¼ cup dessicated coconut, optional
50ml/2 fl oz/¼ cup agave syrup (see page 49)
40g/1½oz/¼ cup chopped hazelnuts

1 Slice the bananas into bite-size chunks and insert lolly sticks into each one. Place in a covered, freezer proof dish and freeze for 2 hours.
2 Enjoy as they are, or dip in hazelnuts, coconut or syrup – or all three.

Dairy-Free Chocolate Rice Pudding
Serves 4

500ml/18 fl oz/2½ cups soya milk
3 tbsp clear honey
a pinch of sea salt
220g/73/4oz/1⅓ cups pudding rice
½ tsp alcohol free natural vanilla essence
80g/3¼oz dairy-free dark chocolate pieces
110ml/4floz/½ cup soya cream
1 tsp cinnamon, optional

1 Place the milk, honey and sea salt in a saucepan and bring to the boil. Add the rice and cook for 20 minutes, stirring.
2 Stir in the vanilla essence.
3 Divide the mixture between 4 serving bowls and insert the chocolate pieces into the middle of each one and leave to

melt. Pour the soya cream over each pudding and sprinkle with cinammon

Dairy-free snacks

All the gluten-free snacks listed at the end of Chapter 4 (see page 60) are also suitable for a dairy-free diet. Make sure that you select a dairy-free dip for the crudités, however. In addition to the aforementioned snacks, you may wish to try some of the following:

Granola A breakfast cereal made from crunchy oats combined with other grains, nuts, seeds and berries. Some may contain milk, so check the ingredients listing carefully. You can eat granola as a dry snack. Add a quantity of the cereal to a suitable bag and carry it with you.

Soy nuts These are made from roasted soya beans.

Banana chips Made from deep-fried bananas and often coated with sugar or honey.

Both granola and banana chips are high-calorie snacks, so eat them in moderation!

7

Candida – Is yeast overgrowth the root of your weight regulation problems?

Imagine if you will, a type of yeast that lives within the digestive system of all humans. It doesn't normally cause any problems as long as the conditions to keep it in check are right. However, given the right conditions, it can change. Like a prisoner, suddenly given the opportunity to make his escape, Candida (*Candida albicans* but I will call it Candida for short) can migrate outside the digestive system and begin to proliferate in different parts of the body. When this happens it can cause no end of problems. Candida is a strain of yeast that lives quite happily within the digestive system. Normally, it doesn't cause any problems because certain factors keep it within the boundaries of the digestive tract.

One such factor is the presence of so-called healthy bacteria in the gut. These are the 'good guys!' Healthy bacteria with strange-sounding names such as *Lactobacillus acidophilus* and *Bifido bifidum* help keep the yeast in check by competing with it for food and territory. But what happens when these bacteria are depleted, or the body's immune system is compromised in some other way? The answer is an overgrowth of Candida within the digestive system, known as candidiasis. Depletion of the friendly bacteria in the gut is a little like removing the prison warders from a prison – all hell would break loose! With no controls to keep the Candida in check it begins to proliferate and the effects can be systemic; not only this but it begins to alter its form and starts to set down root-like structures known as mycelium. These structures penetrate the lining of the intestine resulting in perforations in the gut wall. Normally, the gut wall is porous because it has to allow food particles to be absorbed into the bloodstream. However, once the Candida begins to penetrate the gut wall, these holes are made bigger, resulting in a condition known as 'leaky gut' syndrome. When this happens, larger food particles such as proteins can pass through the gut and enter the bloodstream, resulting in the immune system (which is always on the lookout for foreign invaders) recognising these larger particles as enemies. An immune response is therefore invoked by the body and often paves the way for the development of food allergies and intolerances.

The immune system is usually capable of directing specialised cells to the site of a yeast infection to destroy it. However, what if a person's immune system is depleted, perhaps due to an unhealthy lifestyle? This makes him or her vulnerable to candidiasis. Other factors that can increase susceptibility are:

- *Over-use of antibiotics:* These destroy the micro-organisms they were designed to eliminate; however, they also destroy the healthy bacteria in your gut.
- *Over-consumption of refined foods:* Foods such as white flour, white rice, sugar and fats tend to overload the body with toxins, resulting in an over-stressed immune

system. They also change the pH (acidity or alkalinity) of the gut, making conditions more favourable for yeast overgrowth. What's more, yeasts just love sugar! Put sugar with yeast and it ferments, producing lots of toxic end products. When we eat refined carbohydrates in the form of sugars and flour, we give the yeast the fuel it needs to proliferate.

- *Increased use of steroid medication:* Medication such as this may suppress the immune system, resulting in weakened defences.

- *Low-level antibiotics and steroids in the food chain:* Those who consume animal products such as commercially produced meats (except lamb), eggs and dairy foods are likely to be ingesting steroids and antibiotics given to livestock to prevent disease (often, due to unfavourable living conditions, this is more prevalent) and promote faster growth. Low-level intake of these substances over many years may have an adverse affect on the body's ability to control Candida.

- *Increasing use of Non-Steroidal Anti-Inflammatory Drugs (NSAIDs):* Available over the counter, these are being used for common problems such as joint aches, period pain and other painful conditions. Like antibiotics, they can adversely affect our friendly bacteria, paving the way for Candida to gain ground.

- *Widespread use of steroid medication:* Another principal cause of yeast infections, these drugs have a powerful anti-inflammatory effect in the body. However, their long-term use can have an immuno-suppressant effect. A weakened immune system is less capable of defending the body against yeast infections. That's why some asthma sufferers develop thrush (a type of yeast infection) in their mouths as a result of regular use of steroid-based inhalers. Moreover, it's worth remembering that both Hormone Replacement Therapy (HRT) and the contraceptive pill are forms of steroid treatment. Therefore, women who take these forms of medication also tip the balance in favour of yeast overgrowth.

Bearing in mind all these adverse influences upon the body, it's hardly surprising that candidiasis has reached almost epidemic proportions and yet it rarely receives recognition from conventional doctors. As with food intolerances, yeast overgrowth can cause a multitude of health conditions including weight-gain, which I will discuss later in this chapter. The following health conditions can often be caused by candidiasis:

- *Digestive system:* Irritable Bowel Syndrome (IBS), constipation, abdominal pain, nausea, bloating, flatulence, belching, indigestion, heartburn, mucous in the stools, bad breath, dry mouth, mouth ulcers, oral thrush, rectal itching, food allergies and intolerances, weight regulation problems.
- *Skin:* Athlete's foot, fungal nail infections, acne, ringworm, psoriasis, eczema, urticaria (nettle rash), itching, tendency to bruise.
- *Urinary system:* Frequent urge to urinate, burning sensation, inflammation.
- *Reproductive system:* Vaginal discharge, thrush, itchiness, vaginal burning.
- *Eyes, ears, nose and throat:* Post-nasal drip, catarrh, frequent sore throats, mucous congestion, sinus pain,

itchy nose, laryngitis, loss of voice, 'glue' ear in children, ear infections, dizziness, spots in front of the eyes, recurrent eye infections, watery eyes.

- *Respiratory system:* Recurring bronchial infections such as bronchitis, tightness in the chest, wheezing and asthma.
- *Musculo-skeletal system:* Muscle weakness and aches, swollen joints, painful joints.
- *Central nervous system:* Numbness, tingling, depression, mental 'fogginess', a feeling of being 'spaced out', poor concentration, irritability, mood swings, anxiety attacks, panic attacks, drowsiness.
- *Circulatory system:* Extreme coldness especially hands and feet, inability to keep warm.
- *Immune system:* Frequent infections, susceptibility to M.E. (chronic fatigue syndrome) and auto-immune disorders when the immune system attacks the body's own tissues, such as rheumatoid arthritis and lupus.
- *General:* Lethargy, low energy, weight problems.

Kate's story

Years ago, when I first became involved in food intolerance testing, a young lady booked in for a test. When she arrived at the clinic I remember thinking she looked very healthy. In reality, this was far from the truth for she informed me that she was suffering from digestive problems. She also told me that she was suffering from a condition that affected the muscles in her body. Such was the seriousness of her condition that if she ran to catch a bus, she wouldn't know if her legs would suddenly give way. As if that wasn't bad enough, she was afraid to pick up her sister's baby in case she might suddenly lose control of the muscles in her arms.

Kate had to travel to an Oxford clinic to undergo tests on her muscles. Doctors there had been monitoring her condition for some time, but one thing was certain: she wasn't getting any better.

When she arrived to be tested that day, I was open-minded about what the outcome would be. However, I wasn't too surprised when all of the indications pointed towards a yeast overgrowth. Nevertheless, just to be sure, I asked her to fill in a Candida questionnaire. The answers on this questionnaire are given a score and the higher the number of points scored in relation to your responses to the questions, the greater the likelihood that you are suffering from candidiasis. When I calculated Kate's score she was off the scale! There was no doubt in my mind that she was suffering from yeast overgrowth. I was convinced that this was the cause of her digestive problems but what about the muscle condition? I had my suspicions that her systemic muscle weakness could be linked with the Candida problem, but I don't think I mentioned it at the time.

The first thing she needed to do was to follow an anti-Candida diet and in addition to this, I advised her to take specific herbal anti-fungal supplements. Basically, the diet deprives the yeast of its favourite foods: sugar, refined carbohydrates, fermented foods such as vinegar and alcoholic beverages and mould-growing foods such as cheese and nuts as well as foods that are part of the fungal family such as mushrooms. So, by following this strict diet, the yeast is being starved into submission. What's more, the anti-fungal supplement, which consists of herbal and other natural ingredients known to destroy Candida, is taken alongside the diet. The end result is a double-whammy! The yeast is starved of the foods that help it to thrive while at the same time it is destroyed by the action of the anti-fungal agents. There are drugs that also have an anti-fungal effect but most nutritional therapists and naturopaths prefer to use natural alternatives since these are far less likely to have any adverse side effects.

The big change

To her credit, Kate stuck rigidly to the diet and began to notice positive changes in the first two weeks. First, her digestive symptoms cleared up. She was delighted about that because prior to following the programme, her symptoms were causing her much distress. Even though she was feeling much better, I strongly advised her to carry on with the diet because Candida can easily return if old eating habits begin to creep back in. Secretly, I hoped that she might start to show some signs of improvement with her muscle condition. The big improvement that she experienced gave her the motivation needed to carry on with the diet. This was just as well, for what happened next was astonishing, even to me.

Four or five weeks into the programme, Kate noticed that she had more energy. Instead of returning home after a hard day's work and collapsing in a heap on the sofa, she began to start preparing the evening meal for herself and her partner. She also noticed that her muscles were starting to feel different and she dared to wonder if she might be feeling a little stronger. When the time came for her to return to the clinic in Oxford for her periodic tests, she decided to take her food intolerance test results with her to show the doctors. They were very sceptical about their validity but after conducting several tests, they couldn't deny the truth: her muscles were showing definite signs of improvement. They even gave her the go ahead to try for a family.

From that point on Kate continued to improve. She followed my advice and bought a cross-training machine which she used daily at home. This accelerated the improvement in her muscles. Needless to say, she was delighted with her new state of wellbeing and freedom from illness. The only problem she had was that she began to crave fruit, which she had had to omit from her diet because the fruit sugars feed the yeast. In view of this I suggested that she should re-introduce two pieces of fruit each day to see how she responded. At first she was fine, but after another week or so, she phoned in a distressed state. She had some recurrence of her digestive symptoms. When I asked her if she was still eating the fruit, she said she was. The only thing she'd added into her diet was fruit juice. I explained to her that this contained too much sugar at this stage and that it was feeding the yeast. When she eliminated the fruit juice from her diet, the symptoms disappeared again.

Kate continued to thrive and do well on the diet. Eventually she was able to re-introduce some of the foods she had had to avoid but she was always careful not to get back into her old bad eating patterns. She was a little concerned about her continual weight loss on the diet, but I explained that this was normal and she should not to worry about it because after a while this would level out. I was delighted to see Kate recently, this being several years after the amazing turnaround in her health. She was happy to inform me that she now had two healthy children.

The story of Kate serves to illustrate how far-reaching the effects of yeast overgrowth can be on the body. As with food intolerances, it leads to the question of how many people there are in the world suffering from common health conditions that might respond to some basic changes to their diet and lifestyle.

How candidiasis can stop you shedding the pounds!

One of the ways in which Candida can result in an inability to lose excess pounds is the effect it has on your blood sugar levels. The presence of Candida overgrowth will result in sugar cravings, so to satisfy the cravings you eat sugary foods or refined carbohydrates such as white bread, white pasta and white rice. Refined carbohydrates are rapidly turned into sugar by the body, thus feeding the yeast. Eating these foods gives you an upsurge in blood sugar followed by a dip in energy, after which you crave more of the same type of foods. When you get into this type of eating pattern you are more likely to put on excess weight and you certainly will find it nigh on impossible to lose the pounds.

In addition to its influence on blood sugar levels, Candida also interferes with digestion. As with food intolerances, it appears that a yeast overgrowth can interfere with the metabolic rate as well as the body's ability to absorb nutrients from food. All these factors can result in weight regulation problems. Finally, Candida can increase one's propensity to develop allergies and intolerances, which can result in weight gain as you'll know from reading the earlier chapters in this book. Candida sufferers invariably report that they experience significant weight loss on an anti-Candida programme.

Another aspect of food cravings that can make you fat

Avoiding refined carbohydrates not only feeds Candida, it may further encourage a different kind of food craving that can make you overweight. This type of craving is fuelled by the body's need to eat greater quantities of food because refined carbohydrates and other junk foods don't supply enough of the nutrients required for your body to function properly. These types of foods have a 'double whammy' effect because they are a poor source of the important vitamins and minerals that your body needs to function normally. In fact, they are classed as 'anti-nutrients' because your body actually uses up vitamins and minerals in order to digest them. When this happens you end up craving more and more food to feed your cells what they need. Of course when this happens you can be sure of one thing: all those extra calories get stored up as fat! The answer is to replace junk food with nutrient-packed healthy food. In this way, not only do you not feed the Candida, you also satisfy the nutrient demands of your cells thus helping to break the vicious cycle of eating excessive amounts of food in a vain attempt to provide enough nutrients for your body's needs.

The Anti-Candida Diet and 'die-off' reactions

When the combined action of the diet and anti-fungal remedy begin to take effect, the yeast starts to be destroyed. This usually results in so-called yeast 'die-off' which is, of course, a good thing because it proves that the programme is working. However, when the yeasts get destroyed in this way, they give off a number of toxins that can make you feel nauseated and off-colour. The toxins produced by the yeasts place an extra burden on an already hard-worked liver, which may struggle to detoxify the toxins before the body attempts to void them to the outside of the body. This is why it's a good idea to consult a reputable qualified practitioner to guide you through the programme (see Useful Information, page 30 to find out how to contact a practitioner near you). If you live outside the UK, then seek advice from a recognised national organisation that will provide you with similar information.

Anti-fungal supplements

There are many natural products that possess anti-fungal and anti-bacterial qualities – for example, garlic and onions. These everyday foods are a useful addition to the diet because they do help to keep Candida at bay. However, for someone already suffering from a Candida problem, it's a good idea to take an anti-fungal supplement. These supplements often include caprylic acid (a natural derivative from coconuts that has an anti-fungal action), artemesia and grapefruit seed extract. Grapefruit seed extract may be used on its own towards the end of the anti-Candida programme and can be very useful in finally killing off the yeast overgrowth. Use three or four drops in water twice daily; it has effective anti-fungal and anti bacterial properties.

CAUTION!
Anti-fungals are not recommended if you are pregnant or trying to become pregnant.

Foods to avoid on an Anti-Candida Diet

The following foods must be strictly avoided on an Anti-Candida Diet:

- *Sugar:* In all its forms, sugar must be strictly avoided. The word 'sugar' also includes foods that contain sugar such as biscuits, ice cream, chocolate, puddings, soft drinks such as squash and fizzy drinks. Remember, sugar is also added to many everyday foods such as tomato ketchup and packaged foods so always check the list of ingredients.

- *Refined carbohydrates:* These include all flour from wheat and other grains that have been processed. Therefore, you must avoid white flour and anything made from it, including bread, cakes, biscuits, pasta, macaroni and spaghetti. Add to this list cornflour and any breakfast cereals that are made of (or contain) refined cereals – for example, cornflakes. The simplest approach is just to select wholegrain foods such as wholegrain rice, wholewheat bread, 100% wholewheat pasta, spaghetti, etc. Avoid granary flour and granary bread. A lot of people are fooled into thinking it is wholewheat whereas it's really made from white flour that has been coloured with malt.

- *Yeast:* This includes all forms of yeast such as baker's yeast (found in baked goods like bread, pitta breads, cakes and biscuits), breadcrumb-coated foods, brewer's yeast (found in alcoholic beverages such as wines, beers and spirits), monosodium glutamate, gravies and sauces that include yeast in the ingredients, Bovril, Marmite, Brewer's yeast tablets, vitamin tablets (unless yeast-free is stated on the label) and savoury snacks containing yeast as a flavouring.

- *Fermented foods:* This includes vinegars (although some experts allow cider vinegar, depending upon how you react to it), alcoholic beverages, soy sauce, sourdough bread and foods that contain fermented ingredients – for example, pickles, ketchup, salad cream, mayonnaise, etc.

- *Dairy products:* Exclude milk as it contains sugar in the form of lactose. Also, cheeses as these contain moulds, especially blue cheese. Natural (unsweetened) yoghurt, butter and cottage cheese are permitted, however.
- *Malted products:* Malt is often added to foods as flavouring. Watch out for cereals which sometimes have added malt or malt extract – for example, cornflakes, some crispbreads and malted drinks.
- *Fresh fruit:* This is usually excluded for the first 3–4 weeks of the programme and only re-introduced in small amounts to begin with. Avoid stewed fruit and fruit purées. Fresh fruit also tends to attract moulds that live on the skins of such fruits as grapes, plums and apples. Avoid especially fruit juice as this is highest in fruit sugar (fructose).
- *Dried fruit:* Dried fruit of all kinds contains high levels of fruit sugar so avoid sultanas, raisins, dates, apricots, figs, etc.
- *Smoked and cured foods:* Examples include smoked or cured fish, meats of all kinds, ham and bacon.
- *Nuts:* These tend to attract moulds. However, you can use freshly cracked nuts. The exception to this is peanuts, even in their shells, as they contain a high level of mould. Also avoid peanut butter.
- *Mushrooms:* Avoid these as they are related to moulds (fungi).
- *Tea and coffee:* These contain stimulants that encourage candidiasis. Even decaffeinated coffee and tea contain other stimulants, so avoid them too.

- *Hot spicy foods:* Thought to destroy healthy bacteria in the gut and are therefore to be avoided.
- *Preservatives:* These are often derived from yeasts (citric acid is a good example).
- *Artificial sweeteners:* There is some evidence to suggest that artificial sweeteners may also feed yeasts. Aside from this, most natural health practitioners advise people to avoid them since they are thought to be a causative factor linked with a variety of health conditions.

Now for the good news!

Having read about the foods that you must avoid, you could be forgiven for thinking that there is nothing left for you to eat. Well, don't despair because there are still many delicious foods for you to enjoy:

- *Soya or rice milk:* These are good alternatives to ordinary milk. Look out for the brands that are unsweetened, though.
- *Cottage cheese:* Can be eaten on its own or spread onto rice cakes, etc. It also makes a good filling for baked potatoes.
- *Yeast-free soda breads:* These are fine but you must choose the ones made with wholegrains such as wholewheat and not refined flours.
- *Rice cakes:* Plain or one of the flavoured varieties (avoid those flavoured with yeast or malt). Good spread with cottage cheese or hummus.
- *Oat cakes:* Again, make sure they're made with 100% wholegrain oats. Choose those that don't contain malt.
- *Butter:* This can be used for cooking as well as a spread.
- *Margarine:* Avoid brands containing hydrogenated fats or citric acid.
- *Natural yoghurt:* Delicious with seeds such as sesame, or

sunflower. Alternatively, sweeten with a little FOS (Fructo-oligo-saccharides see below).

- *Meat and poultry:* Where possible, select free-range organic. Commercially reared animals usually contain antibiotics and steroids, although lamb and wild game is less likely to present a problem.
- *Fish:* Avoid smoked and/or breaded fish. Otherwise, all types are fine.
- *Breakfast cereals:* Not all breakfast cereals are bad news! I often recommend that clients try making their own muesli using a combination of wholegrains to which you can add seeds such as sesame or pumpkin. You can enjoy your cereal with soya or rice milk. Also, try making homemade porridge using whole oats or buy a ready-made breakfast cereal made from 100% wholegrains (for instance, some organic cornflakes are available that contain no sweeteners and are made from 100% corn and a little salt; choose the wholegrain type, though).
- *Vegetables:* Make use of a wide variety of vegetables including steamed, lightly boiled and stir-fried. Try to have at least one large salad daily and include foods such as onions and garlic, which have natural anti-fungal properties.
- *Avocados:* Nutritious and filling, they can be eaten on their own or sliced and added to salads. You can also make a nice salad and avocado filling for sandwiches. Alternatively, slice the avocado lengthways, remove the stone and fill with hummus or cooked prawns.
- *Pulses:* These include lentils, chickpeas and all kinds of beans. They are great for making dishes such as lentil bakes and onion bhajis.
- *Seeds:* Unlike nuts, these are fine as they don't tend to

attract moulds. There are plenty to choose from, including sesame, sunflower, pumpkin, flax and hemp seeds.

- *Freshly cracked nuts:* With the exception of peanuts, these are a good addition to your diet and, like seeds, a good source of healthy fats.
- *Lemons:* Along with avocadoes, this is the only fruit allowed. Lemon juice is great for making salad dressings and it can be used to make a hot drink; sweetened with a little FOS, see below, if desired.
- *Mild spices:* Make use of spices such as cinnamon, cumin, coriander and turmeric but avoid the hot ones such as chillis.
- *Hot beverages:* These can include herb teas (choose from fennel, chamomile, peppermint, etc.), dandelion coffee (if not flavoured with sugar, e.g. lactose) and rooibosch tea.
- *Herbs:* All kinds of herbs can be used to add interesting flavours to your meals – for example, fresh chopped basil or mint can be sprinkled over salads. Dried herbs may be stirred in to soups or casseroles.
- *Cold drinks:* The best ones are bottled or filtered still or sparkling water. Add ice and slices of lemon to make a refreshing drink.
- *FOS (fructo-oligo-saccharides):* Basically, a sweet-tasting, soluble fibre found in some vegetables and fruits. The good news is that it feeds the beneficial bacteria in the digestive system while yeasts cannot use it. This type of food is referred to as a pre-biotic because it actually feeds healthy bacteria such as *Lactobacillus acidophilus* and *Bifido bifidum*, so helping to maintain or restore the healthy bacteria population, which in turn helps to keep yeast organisms in check. In recent years, an increasing number of food manufacturers are beginning to add FOS

as a pre-biotic to their products. It's not unusual to find it in yoghurts and fruit and cereal bars.

For those Candida sufferers who simply must have something sweet, FOS is the solution: it can be purchased in powdered form and added to yoghurts, cereals and drinks. However, don't expect it to flow and dissolve like ordinary sugar. When added to liquids, it tends to form lumps. Nevertheless, if you stir it enough, it does impart sweetness to whatever food it is mixed with. Be careful when taking it for the first time because even small amounts can cause wind and flatulence due to its action upon the gut flora but this should diminish as your digestive system gets used to it.

A WORD ABOUT THE USE OF NATURAL SWEETENERS THAT DON'T FEED CANDIDA

Some nutritional therapists and naturopaths believe that Candida sufferers should not resort to using FOS as a sugar substitute. Their argument is that this does nothing to help sufferers overcome their sweet tooth. My own feeling on this issue is that some people cope better with the programme if certain concessions are made concerning the use of such sweeteners (not to be confused with artificial sweeteners, which are not allowed). Also, in my experience, after adhering to the anti-Candida diet for some time, the desire for sugary foods as well as refined carbohydrates tends to subside. I have even witnessed how former 'chocoholics' lose their desire to eat chocolate. Bearing this in mind, I have included FOS in the recipes that follow.

Anti-Candida recipes

The big challenge with breakfast dishes is that they're often sweetened. There are, however, plenty of ways to avoid sugar at the start of the day, and the following recipes will give you an idea of the various ways to make a healthy start on an Anti-Candida diet.

Breakfasts

Having read the earlier chapters in this book, you'll know by now that I'm a fan of homemade muesli. The beauty is that you can adapt it according to your specific needs and this principle applies equally when making an anti-Candida version. Here is one example of a muesli free from Candida-feeding ingredients:

Homemade Muesli

In a bowl, mix together the following flaked cereals:
300g/10oz/2 cups rolled oats
300g/10oz/2 cups rye flakes
300g/10oz/2 cups wheat flakes
150g/5oz/1 cup buckwheat flakes

Now add the following seeds:
2 tbsp pumpkin seeds
2 tbsp sesame seeds
3 tbsp shelled hemp seeds

Transfer to an airtight container. Serve with soya or rice milk and sweeten with a little FOS, if desired. The muesli should keep for a couple of weeks if kept in an airtight container.

Millet Porridge
Serves 2–4

225g/8oz/1¼ cups millet
juice of ½ lemon
1 litre/1¾ pints/5 cups water
2 tbsp of sesame seeds

Mix the millet, lemon juice and water in a saucepan and bring to the boil, then simmer for 1 hour. Serve in individual breakfast bowls sprinkled with sesame seeds.

Toast and Seed Butter
Serves 1

2 slices wholewheat yeast-free soda bread (or yeast-free soda rye bread)
50g/2oz sunflower or pumpkin seed butter

Pop the bread in a toaster and when golden brown, spread with the seed butter and serve.

Soya Yoghurt and Hemp Seed Mix
Serves 1

1 small pot (approx 150g/5oz) plain soya yoghurt
1 tbsp shelled hemp seeds
FOS to taste, optional
a pinch of cinnamon

1 Pour the yoghurt into a breakfast bowl and stir in the hemp seeds.
2 Add the FOS, if using, and mix well. Serve sprinkled with cinnamon.

Scrambled Eggs on Wholewheat Yeast-Free Soda Bread
Serves 1–2

2 free-range, preferably organic, eggs
2 tbsp soya or rice milk
1 tbsp butter
2 slices of wholewheat, yeast-free soda bread
freshly ground black pepper
a little sea salt

1 Place the eggs, soya or rice milk in a bowl and beat together well.
2 Gently melt the butter in a saucepan over a medium heat. Add the egg mixture and stir until scrambled to your liking.
3 Toast the bread, layer the scrambled eggs on top, season and serve.

Seed Butter and Sprouted Seeds Sandwich
Serves 1
This is a very nutritious, quick-to-prepare breakfast sandwich.

25g/1oz pumpkin seed butter
2 slices whole rye yeast-free soda bread

25g/1oz/½ cup alfalfa sprouts (or other sprouted seeds of
   your choice)
mineral water or herb tea, to serve

Spread the pumpkin seed butter over the bread and make a
sandwich using the sprouted seeds as the filling. Serve with a
glass of sparkling mineral water and a slice of lemon or
herbal tea.

Natural Bio-Yoghurt with Toasted Sesame Seeds
Serves 1

1 small pot (approx 150g/5oz) plain bio-yoghurt
1 tsp toasted sesame seeds

Place the yoghurt and sesame seeds in a breakfast bowl, mix
together well and serve.

Grilled Tomatoes and 'Cheese' on Toast
Serves 1

2 slices wholewheat yeast-free soda bread
a little butter
1 large tomato, sliced
1 tbsp grated yeast-free, sugar-free and dairy-free cheese such as
   dairy-free Parmesan
Freshly ground black pepper

1 Preheat the grill to medium. Meanwhile, toast the bread in
   the toaster. Spread with butter and cover with tomato

slices. Place under the grill until the tomatoes soften and are cooked through.

2 Remove from the heat, sprinkle with cheese and return to the grill for a few seconds until the cheese begins to melt. Season and serve.

Main meals

Many of the following recipes do not require yeast, sugar or dairy products. Where necessary, I have given substitute ingredients so that you can enjoy some of your favourite dishes even when following the Anti-Candida diet.

Pasta Tuna Bake

Serves 2

Serve with a salad of your choice or with lightly steamed vegetables such as asparagus and broccoli

1 tbsp butter
2 heaped tsp rice flour
225ml/8 fl oz/1 cup soya milk
600g/1lb 5oz/3 cups wholewheat pasta
1 tbsp extra virgin olive oil
1 large onion, (chopped)
1 garlic clove, sliced
1 small can (200g/7oz) of tuna in oil, drained
sea salt
freshly ground black pepper

1 Place the butter in a saucepan and gently melt over low heat. Stir in the rice flour then add the soya milk and stir until the sauce thickens.

2 Meanwhile, heat a large pan of salted water and cook the pasta according to the package directions until tender. In a frying pan heat the olive oil and sauté the onions and garlic until slightly browned.

3 Drain the cooked pasta and add it to the sauce, together with the cooked onions and garlic. Mix well to combine and continue to gently heat.

4 Add the tuna to the pasta and mix thoroughly. Season.

Mild Spicy Chicken
Serves 1

2 tbsp extra virgin olive oil
2 onions, chopped
1 garlic clove, chopped
4 free-range (preferably organic) skinned chicken portions
1 tbsp paprika
150ml/¼ pint/¾ cup yeast-free vegetable stock
a pinch of sea salt
freshly ground black pepper
1 small pot (approx 150g/5oz) plain natural or soya yoghurt
lightly cooked vegetables such as pak choi, cabbage and carrots and
    wholegrain rice, to serve

1 Heat the oil and gently fry the onions and garlic in a large frying pan for a few minutes until golden. Add the chicken and paprika and cook for a further few minutes, turning once.

2 Mix in the vegetable stock, add the seasoning and simmer for 25–30 minutes. When cooked, stir in the yoghurt and serve with lightly cooked vegetables or wholegrain rice.

Vegetable Casserole
Serves 4

a little butter for frying
2 garlic cloves, chopped
1 large onion, chopped
1 tbsp extra virgin olive oil
4 medium potatoes, diced
2 courgettes, sliced
1 leek, sliced
1 red pepper, deseeded and chopped
150g/5oz/1 cup fresh or frozen garden peas
¼ cauliflower, chopped
2 carrots, sliced
1 large can (approx 450g/1lb) of chopped tomatoes
225g/8oz/1 cup canned, cooked chickpeas
500ml/18 fl oz/½ cup yeast-free vegetable stock
2 tsp mixed herbs
¼tsp sea salt
freshly ground black pepper

1 Melt the butter in a pan and gently fry the garlic and onion for a few minutes until slightly browned. Meanwhile heat the oil in a large casserole, add the vegetables and fry for about 10 minutes, stirring, to soften.
2 Add the onions, garlic, canned tomatoes and chickpeas. Pour in the stock, sprinkle with herbs and seasoning then bring to the boil. Reduce the heat and leave to simmer for about 30 minutes. This is delicious served with wholewheat yeast-free soda bread drizzled with olive oil.

Vegetables and Fried Rice
Serves 4

100g/3½oz/½ cup wholegrain rice
3 tbsp extra virgin olive oil
2 garlic cloves, chopped
1 large onion, chopped
5 cobs of baby corn, sliced
3 tomatoes, sliced
50g/2oz/½ cup cooked garden peas
1 courgette, chopped
1 red or yellow pepper, deseeded and chopped
50g 12oz French beans, chopped
50g/2oz/1 cup mixed fresh herbs such as chives, basil and mint,
    chopped
1 tsp pumpkin seed oil

1 Cook the rice in a saucepan of boiling salted water according to the package directions until tender. Drain well and rinse under cold water; drain again.
2 Heat a wok and add the olive oil to heat through. Add the garlic and onion; stir-fry for about 30 seconds. Add the remaining vegetables and stir-fry for 2–3 minutes.
3 Add the rice to the mixture and stir-fry for 1–2 minutes. Drizzle with the herbs and pumpkin seed oil and serve.

Tuna Fish Cakes
Makes 4–6

450g/1lb potatoes, quartered
¼ tsp sea salt

freshly ground black pepper
1 small can (approx 200g/7oz) tuna in brine or oil
100g/4oz/½ cup grated onion
2 tbsp finely chopped fresh parsley
2 tbsp wholewheat flour
1 tbsp extra virgin olive oil, for frying
Lemon juice

1   Place the potatoes in a pan of boiling salted water. Bring to
    the boil and then simmer until tender, about 15–20
    minutes. Season and mash thoroughly.
2   Add the tuna to the mashed potatoes and mix well.
    Combine with the grated onion and parsley and shape
    into patties.
3   Lightly coat both sides in flour. Heat the olive oil in a
    frying pan and lightly fry the fishcakes on both sides until
    crisp and golden brown. Sprinkle with lemon juice. Serve
    on their own or with salad or cooked vegetables such as
    cauliflower and peas.

Mixed Vegetable Soup
Serves 2

1 tbsp olive oil
2 large onions, chopped
1 garlic clove, sliced
5 tsp tomato paste (without citric acid)
1.2 litres/2 pints/6 cups yeast-free vegetable stock
2 courgettes, sliced
3 large carrots, sliced
225g/8oz/2 cups shredded white cabbage

150g/5oz/2 cups broccoli florets
100g/31/2oz/½ cup split lentils
½ tsp sea salt
freshly ground black pepper
1 tsp turmeric
wholewheat yeast-free soda bread or the rye bread, to serve

1 Heat the oil in a saucepan and lightly fry the onions and garlic until softened. Stir in the tomato paste.
2 Add the stock and all the vegetables. Continue to heat for a further 5–6 minutes.
3 Add the lentils, seasoning and turmeric. Cover and bring to the boil, then reduce the heat and leave to simmer for 35 minutes. Serve with wholewheat yeast-free soda bread or the rye bread version.

Carrot, Swede and Potato Mash
Serves 2
For a great combination, serve with steamed or grilled fish.

4 large potatoes, cut into quarters
1 medium swede, diced
4 carrots, sliced
2 tbsp butter
½ tsp sea salt
freshly ground black pepper
1 small pot (approx 150g/5oz) of soya or plain natural yoghurt

1 Place the potatoes, swede and carrots in a pan of salted water. Bring to the boil and then leave simmer for 20 minutes until the vegetables are thoroughly cooked.

2 Drain thoroughly. Add the butter, seasoning and yoghurt; mash until smooth and creamy.

Ratatouille

Serves 4

This is a great combination with wholegrain rice or a baked potato.

3 courgettes, diced
2 aubergines, diced
1 tbsp extra virgin olive oil
1 large onion, chopped
2 garlic cloves, sliced
2 green peppers, deseeded and sliced
1 large can (approx 450g/1lb) chopped tomatoes (without citric acid)
2 tbsp tomato paste (no citric acid)
1 tbsp mixed fresh or dried herbs such as chives, basil and coriander
½ tsp sea salt
freshly ground black pepper

1 Place the courgettes and aubergines in a colander and sprinkle with the salt. Cover and leave for 25 minutes. Rinse and drain.
2 Heat the oil in a large saucepan. Gently fry the onion and garlic for 4–5 minutes. Add the peppers, courgettes and aubergines. Mix well, then fry for 5 minutes.
3 Stir in the chopped tomatoes and tomato paste. Cover and then gently simmer for a further 30 minutes.
4 Add the herbs and seasoning; mix well before serving.

Salads

Grated Root Salad and Avocado

Serves 2

This salad is very good for an anti-Candida diet since it contains onions, garlic, lemon juice and olive oil, all of which have anti-fungal properties.

2 large carrots, grated
¼ head celeriac, grated
1 medium beetroot, grated
1 garlic clove, finely sliced
1 red onion, finely sliced
1 tbsp sunflower seeds
juice of 1 lemon
1 tbsp extra virgin olive oil
1 large avocado
1 fresh mint sprig

1 Place the grated vegetables, sliced garlic and onion and sunflower seeds in a large salad bowl and mix well to combine.
2 Stir in the lemon juice and the olive oil.
3 Slice the avocado in half, remove the stone, peel and cut lengthways into slices.
4 Arrange the slices of avocado over the top and garnish with mint leaves to serve.

Tomato and Cottage Cheese Salad
Serves 2

450g/lb/2½ cups tomatoes, thinly sliced
2 tbsp fresh chopped chives
1 tbsp fresh chopped basil
1 tbsp olive oil
a pinch of sea salt
freshly ground black pepper
1 large pot (approx 350g/12oz) of cottage cheese

Arrange the tomatoes on a shallow platter. Sprinkle the herbs over the top and drizzle with olive oil. Season and serve with the cottage cheese.

Rice and Mixed Bean Salad
Serves 2

1 onion, chopped
75g/3oz/½ cup cooked red kidney beans
75g/3oz/½ cup cooked haricot beans
½ cucumber, chopped
1 courgette, chopped
50g/2oz/½ cup black pitted olives
450gg/8oz/2 cups wholegrain rice cooked
2 tbsp olive oil
juice of 1 lemon
a pinch of sea salt
wholewheat or yeast-free soda bread or rice cakes, to serve

1 Mix together the onions, beans, cucumber and courgette in a bowl. Halve the olives and add to the mixture.

2 Add the vegetables with the brown rice and mix thoroughly.
3 Whisk together the olive oil, lemon juice and sea salt in a jug; pour over the salad and toss to combine. Serve with bread or rice cakes.

Chicken Salad
Serves 4

2 tbsp olive oil
2 organic skinless chicken breasts
150g/5oz green beans
8 cherry tomatoes, halved
1 medium carrot, grated
1 tbsp olive oil, for frying
freshly ground black pepper
a pinch of sea salt
juice of 1 lemon
50g/2oz/2 cups baby spinach

1 Gently heat the oil in a frying pan, add the chicken breasts and cook thoroughly on both sides.
2 Meanwhile, steam the green beans until tender and refresh in cold water. In a bowl, mix the beans with the tomatoes and carrot.
3 Place the oil, seasoning and lemon juice in a bowl and whisk until well combined.
4 Layer the salad onto plates. Slice the cooked chicken into thin strips and arrange over the top. Drizzle with dressing, garnish with baby spinach and serve.

Tuna, Egg and Mixed Salad

Serves 2

The use of cold-pressed rapeseed oil for the dressing adds a nutty flavour to the salad. It is also a good source of Omega 3 and Omega 6 essential fatty acids.

175g/6oz/3 cups shredded iceberg lettuce
2 tomatoes, chopped
1 red pepper, deseeded and chopped
3 spring onions, trimmed and sliced
200g/7oz/2 cups shredded cabbage

1 small can (approx 200g/7oz) of tuna in oil
2 free-range eggs, hard-boiled and quartered
juice of 1 lemon
freshly ground black pepper
2 tbsp cold pressed rapeseed oil
50g/2oz/1 cup baby spinach

1 Place lettuce, tomatoes, red pepper, spring onions and cabbage in a salad bowl; mix well. Stir in the tuna and chopped eggs.

2 Whisk together the lemon juice, pepper and rapeseed oil in a bowl. Pour the dressing over the salad and toss together to combine. Garnish with baby spinach and serve.

Wholewheat Macaroni and Butter Bean Salad

Serves 2

450g/1lb/3 cups cooked and drained wholewheat macaroni
225g/8oz/2½ cups cooked butter beans

3 sticks celery, trimmed and chopped

I red onion, chopped

I red or yellow pepper, deseeded and diced

65g/2I/2oz/½ cup sunflower seeds

6 tbsp olive oil

3 tbsp lemon juice

a pinch of sea salt

freshly ground black pepper

4 iceberg lettuce leaves, rinsed and patted dry

1 In a large bowl, combine the macaroni and the butter beans. Add the celery, onion, pepper and sunflower seeds; mix well.

2 Whisk together the oil, lemon juice and seasoning in a bowl and mix well. Pour over the salad and macaroni mixture and toss well to combine.

3 Line a serving bowl with lettuce leaves, add the mixture into a bowl on top and serve.

Potato, Mixed Vegetable and Chicken Salad
Serves 2

I tbsp olive oil

I tbsp lemon juice or cider vinegar

450g/1lb/3 cups cooked and diced new potatoes

I can (450g/1lb) fresh or frozen peas, cooked and drained

I red onion, chopped

I carrot, grated

175ml/6 fl oz/⅔ cup plain soya yoghurt

a pinch of sea salt

freshly ground black pepper

300g/10oz/2 cups cooked chicken pieces
1 bunch of watercress

1 Whisk together the oil and lemon juice or cider vinegar in a bowl and pour over the diced potatoes.
2 In another bowl, combine the peas, onions and grated carrot with the yoghurt and seasoning; add to the potato mixture and mix well.
3 Arrange on a serving platter and pile the cooked chicken pieces on top. Garnish with sprigs of watercress and serve.

Desserts

The following desserts are just as delicious as many conventional versions, and the imaginative use of alternative ingredients such as FOS and coconut make them ideal for Candida sufferers.

Coconut Yoghurt

Serves 1

1 small pot (approx 150g/5oz) plain bio-yoghurt
1 tbsp dessicated coconut
a few drops of alcohol-free natural vanilla essence
1 tsp sunflower seeds

In a bowl thoroughly mix the yoghurt, dessicated coconut and vanilla essence together. Sprinkle with sunflower seeds and serve.

Yoghurt Ice Lollies
Makes 6

1 large pot plain natural yoghurt or soya (yoghurt approx 450g/1lb)
1 tsp of FOS powder

In a bowl, whisk together the yoghurt and FOS powder. Pour the mixture into a 6-capacity lolly mould and place in the freezer. Remove when the lollies are frozen.

Carob-Flavoured Yoghurt
Serves 1

Carob powder is derived from carob beans, which grow on trees in countries such as Spain with warm climates. Their chocolate-like taste can be a welcome addition to an anti-Candida diet but only as an occasional treat as they contain some natural sugars.

1 small pot (150g/5oz) plain natural or soya yoghurt
1 tsp carob powder
a few drops of alcohol-free natural vanilla essence
a pinch of FOS, optional
1 tsp shelled hemp or sunflower seeds

Pour the yoghurt into a bowl and add the carob powder, vanilla essence and FOS, if desired; mix thoroughly. Sprinkle with shelled hemp or sunflower seeds and serve.

Carob and Vanilla Custard

Serves 2

The custard powder that we can buy from the shops is based upon cornflour, which is refined, and therefore not recommended for an anti-Candida diet. Fortunately it's possible to use fine maize meal, which is the unrefined version of cornflour.

I tbsp fine maize meal
300ml/½ pint soya or rice milk
I free-range, preferably organic, egg
I tbsp carob powder
¼ tsp alcohol-free natural vanilla essence

1 In a bowl, mix together the maize meal and a little soya or rice milk until a paste is formed. Beat in the egg.
2 Gently heat the remaining milk in a saucepan. Pour over the mixture in the bowl. Return to the saucepan and stir until the mixture starts to thicken. Remove from the heat while continuing to stir until the custard thickens.
3 Add the carob powder and vanilla essence, mix well and serve.

Carob-Coated Seeds

Serves 2

I tbsp butter
2 tbsp carob powder
I tsp alcohol-free natural vanilla essence
150g/5oz/I cup mixed seeds (sunflower, pumpkin, sesame and shelled hemp)

1 Melt the butter in a saucepan over gentle heat and stir in the carob powder and vanilla essence.

2 Sprinkle in the seeds and coat well with the carob mixture. Arrange on greaseproof paper and place in the refrigerator to set for about two hours. They will keep for several days in an air-tight container.

Rice Pudding

Serves 4

Serve hot or chill in the refrigerator and eat as a cold pudding.

325g/11oz/1¾ cups wholegrain rice
1.2 litres/2 pints/6 cups unsweetened soya milk
juice of 1 lemon
1 tsp cinnamon powder
2 tsp FOS powder

Place all the ingredients in a large saucepan. Bring to the boil and then lower the heat and simmer for around 35 minutes or until the rice has softened.

Yoghurt Milkshake

Serves 2

Large pot (450g/1lb of plain bio-yoghurt or soya yoghurt
1 tbsp shelled hemp seeds
½ tsp alcohol-free natural vanilla essence
1 tsp FOS
4 ice cubes

Place all of the ingredients except the ice cubes in a liquidiser and blend until smooth. Add the ice cubes and blend again. Serve at once.

Seed Butter Toastie
Serves 1
This toasted sandwich is sweetened with FOS and is a nice contrast to the savoury version.

2 slices wholewheat or whole rye yeast-free soda bread
30g/1¼oz butter
50g/2oz nut butter such as almond
1 tps FOS

Coat one side of each slice of bread with butter and the other side with nut butter; sprinkle with FOS. Make a sandwich with the buttered sides of bread facing outwards and place in a toasted sandwich maker. After about 5 minutes, remove from the toaster, cut in half and serve.

Snacks
The following snacks are suitable for an anti-Candida diet (some of the options have also been listed in previous chapters):

- *Homemade popcorn:* This is made very quickly and easily at home. Simply fry the corn in a frying pan until popped and season with a little sea salt, or sweeten with FOS.
- *Raw vegetables* such as carrots, cauliflower and celery can be carried with you in a resealable bag or airtight container. You can also include a dip such as hummus.

- *Seeds:* A great snack that helps stave off hunger in between meals. Good choices are pumpkin, sesame, shelled hemp and sunflower seeds.
- *Oat cakes or rice cakes:* Spread with a little butter or seed butter.
- *Avocados:* Not normally thought of as a snack, however they are very nutritious and sustaining.
- *Soya or natural yoghurt* Sweetened with FOS or served plain, add your favourite seeds as a variation.
- *Sandwiches made from whole wheat or whole rye yeast-free soda bread and your choice of filling:* For example, pumpkin seed butter, tahina (a spread made from sesame seeds) or tuna.
- *Corn chips:* Choose only those made from 100% corn and ensure they are free from forbidden additives such as dairy ingredients. The organic types that are available from some supermarkets and health food shops are often the most pure.

8

Other types of intolerances

In the preceding chapters of this book I have dealt with what I sometimes refer to as the 'big four' food intolerances: gluten, wheat, dairy and yeast although the latter can be more of an indicator of yeast overgrowth than just an intolerance as such. Over the years, my involvement with food intolerance testing has given me the opportunity to make certain observations and to draw some interesting conclusions. One thing I noticed in particular was that often clients suffering from any of the 'big four' would be sensitive to other, less recognised ones – for example, any number of fruit or vegetables or maybe certain meats, fish, pulses or beverages such as coffee or wine. Now you may think that this in itself isn't really unusual – after all, we often hear about people who may have an intolerance to a food such as broccoli or strawberries; in fact, you might have such an intolerance yourself. While I would agree that there are plenty of people who suffer from such sensitivities, during the course of my work, I soon began to realise that they were often an offshoot from one or more of the primary intolerances or to put it another way, people who had any of the major four intolerances often tested positive for one or more of the less well known ones. This in itself doesn't seem unusual because if a person's immune system is being compromised by any of the big four, then surely they must be more vulnerable to sensitivities to other foods. In fact, this proved to be a common scenario with many of the clients who consulted me over the years.

Another amazing aspect to this pattern also began to emerge, however. I soon noticed that when someone addressed their intolerance to any of the four principle intolerances, not only did they feel better but they also began to test negative for the other problem foods. This often happened about two or three months into their gluten-free diet (or whatever exclusion diet they were adhering to). Sure enough, when they were re-tested, the same foods they had originally tested positive for no longer seemed to be a problem. So, what was happening? Well, I soon concluded that when someone was intolerant to, let's say wheat, and they excluded it from their diet, this then paved the way for the healing process to take place within their digestive system. Remember, becoming sensitive to something like wheat causes damage and inflammation of the lining of the intestines. I reasoned that by omitting the food that was causing the damage, not only does the digestive system heal itself over time, it also becomes less sensitive to the other foods for which the individual originally tested positive. In other words, it reduces sensitivity to other foods. Obviously this is good news for the individual concerned, being further proof that the programme is working.

Of course, out of all the people being tested, a minority still had a problem with foods that don't fall into the big four category. Often, however, if they excluded those foods from their diet long enough, they would sometimes be able to re-introduce them without any problem. This is in direct contrast to someone who has a food allergy, which usually means that they have to avoid certain foods for life.

TOP TIP!

If you think you might be suffering from an intolerance to a food that doesn't fall into the aforementioned big four category, you would be well advised to have yourself tested anyway. By doing this you may well discover that you are, after all, intolerant to something like gluten, which could be resulting in your tomato intolerance (or whatever else it might be).

Some less major food intolerances

When I say 'less major food intolerances', I'm not really saying that they are uncommon in themselves or that they have less of an impact when compared to more widely recognised foods such as wheat, what I mean is that often these foods don't make the headlines. Let's face it, you don't usually see a newspaper headline stating something like EGG INTOLERANCE ON THE INCREASE Or maybe LETTUCE INTOLERANCE – THE NEW EPIDEMIC. Nevertheless, if you happen to be sensitive to any of these foods, then at best, it can be very inconvenient and somewhat annoying and at worst, sometimes very debilitating. For a start, you have to scrutinise labels to check ingredients and that's not to mention the fact that you may have to look for alternative ingredients when it comes to preparing your own meals. What's more, if you eat any of the foods with which you have a problem, you can suffer just as many health conditions as someone who has an intolerance to any of the aforementioned four major intolerances, including weight control problems. This is because the body still regards whatever you've become sensitive to as a toxin and usually some uncomfortable symptoms will be manifested as a result of this. For example, it's not unusual for clients to say to me: 'Every time I eat cucumber, a few hours later I feel nauseous.' This is clearly an indication that the body is not happy with that particular food. Another example might be someone who has a problem with potatoes because every time they eat them they suffer from mucous congestion and sinus headaches. Of course, once the offending food (or foods) are removed from their diet, then often the symptoms magically disappear.

Watch out for those detox symptoms!

One of the great aspects of my job is that it gives me the opportunity to help people regain control of their health. I truly love to witness how a person can become pro-active in terms of controlling their health, perhaps for the first time in many years. Nevertheless, I have to warn people that sometimes they may feel worse before they get better. I believe this happens because the body is no longer bombarded with the offending food (toxin) and it seizes the opportunity to give itself a 'houseclean'. In other words, your body begins to detoxify itself. When this happens, that skin condition that you associate with eating onions may initially become worse when you eliminate them from your diet. Recently, I came across someone who suffered from blocked-up sinuses as a result of their intolerance to potatoes. After avoiding them for just a few days, he began to suffer from one head cold after another. During that time he started to produce lots of mucous which made him feel miserable. Recognising what was happening, I encouraged him to continue to avoid potatoes. About a week later he telephoned me to say that he no longer had sinus pain and not only that, but his sense of smell (which had been absent for several years) was returning.

Some everyday problem foods

Sometimes I am asked a question such as 'I can't understand why I'm intolerant to cucumber, surely it's mostly water?' In response to this I have to explain that every food has its own unique chemical composition and that the body's immune system is simply 'earmarking' that particular substance (food) as an enemy. This means that any food, no matter how seemingly innocuous it may appear, can cause someone, somewhere, a problem.

Having said this, there are some foods that more commonly cause problems than others. Take a look at the following list of foods: quite frequently, they cause reactions in some people. Wherever possible, I have given a substitute for the food concerned:

- *Eggs:* Allergies to eggs are well known, however egg intolerance is more common than most people think. Try powdered egg substitutes. They are available from some supermarkets and many health food shops.
- *Soya* can be found in lots of food products including some bakery products (e.g. some types of bread), sweets, drinks, ice cream, breakfast cereals, processed meats and margarine. There are, of course, many specialised soya products, the most common being soya milk and cream, tofu and soya meat substitutes. Soya intolerances can be

quite common in both children and adults. Choose alternatives such as rice, almond and oat milks. These can be used as a substitute for soya milk (when you need a milk to add to breakfast cereals, for example). They are also suitable for a variety of recipes.

- *Nuts:* Most people are familiar with nut allergies, especially to peanuts. However, I come across nut intolerances quite a lot. Remember that different nuts or nut products are often added to packaged and canned foods. Since 2005 food label regulations stipulate that manufacturers must state on their labels whether foods contain nuts or nut-based ingredients. This applies to all pre-packaged foods sold in the UK and the European Union. Someone who is intolerant to one type of nut – for example, almonds – may be fine with other nuts such as Brazil nuts. Apart from being careful to scrutinise labels, you can always opt for seeds instead of any nut (or nuts) that you may be sensitive to. Also, choose seed butters instead of nut butter (e.g. sunflower instead of peanut butter).
- *Seeds:* Sometimes I come across a person who is sensitive to seeds such as sunflower or pumpkin. Fortunately, as with nuts, they are usually not intolerant to all of them. If you can eat certain nuts, simply substitute them for the seeds that you have a problem with.
- *Rice:* Now this one may surprise a lot of people because rice isn't usually associated with allergies or intolerances. Interestingly enough, rice allergies and intolerances are much more common in Eastern Asian countries such as Japan, where rice is a staple part of the diet. This seems to mirror what is happening with wheat here in the West, when overexposure to a given food is more likely to result in an over-sensitivity. Provided you are OK with the other

grains (or at least some of them), it is not too hard to avoid rice by simply substituting another grain. But what happens when you are intolerant to all grains, even the non-gluten ones? In such circumstances I usually advise people to make good use of pulses. For example, chickpeas can be used to make flour. Another name for chickpea flour is gram flour and it is used a lot in Indian cookery to make poppadoms, bhajis and other recipes.

- *Fish:* Allergies can cause severe reactions, including anaphylactic shock, in some people. This is when the immune system reacts severely to a specific food such as peanuts and produces large amounts of histamine, which results in swelling of the bodies' tissues. When this happens in the mouth and throat, it can be life threatening. I haven't noticed such severe reactions in people who are intolerant to fish, however. To avoid fish altogether, it's important to read labels. Obviously if a manufacturer states that their product is suitable for vegans or vegetarians, then it must be free from fish or fish products. Bear in mind that it's possible to be intolerant to one type of fish, but not necessarily all fish. This also applies to shellfish.

- *Meat:* As with fish, it's possible to be intolerant to one or two meats, but not necessarily to them all. Sometimes people can be intolerant to more than one type of meat because they're from the same food family – for example, hare and rabbit. Be sure to carefully scrutinise ingredients as meat and meat derivatives are often added to food products. If you don't have a problem with soya, you can use it as a meat substitute. There are also many ready-made soya meat products that you can buy from supermarkets and health food shops. Also, use pulses to make high protein dishes – for example, lentil bakes and chickpea casseroles. It's also a good idea to opt for organic meats whenever possible because they are less likely to contain contaminants such as antibiotics and hormones, which some people can be sensitive to.

- *Fruit and vegetables:* Fortunately, most people are not intolerant to all fruits, although I have come across some cases of this. Also, because fruit is such an important part of your diet, it's a good idea to try and establish which ones you can tolerate and include them in your diet whenever possible. Apart from establishing whether you can eat some fruits, be sure to make up for any lack of fruits with plenty of vegetables. Check labels on products to see if any excluded fruits or their fruit derivatives have been added. As with fruits, most people are not usually intolerant to all vegetables and it's important to establish which ones you can tolerate. Again, try to compensate for any lack of vegetables in your diet by eating more fruits. I would also recommend that you take a good multi-vitamin and mineral supplement from a reputable company (see Useful Information, page 301).

- *Fructose:* Another name for fructose is fruit sugar because it is the main sugar found in fruits. However, don't be misled by the name because it's also present in many vegetables and other foods – for example, carrots and beetroot. Fructose intolerance (sometimes referred to as fructose malabsorption) and Hereditary Fructose Intolerance (HFI) are two distinct metabolic disorders where the body does not tolerate fructose well. Sometimes it is mistakenly referred to in medical terminology as 'fructose allergy', a condition that appears to be unheard of. HFI is a condition due to a lack of a specific chemical in the liver that is needed to break down the fructose.

Fructose malabsorption, on the other hand, more widely referred to as 'fructose intolerance', is much more common than HFI. This is really an inability in the body to absorb fructose through the small intestine. Fructose is normally transported via the wall of the intestine by a specific protein. If this protein is missing, fructose fails to be absorbed and travels to the large intestine. Once there it is fermented by intestinal bacteria and produces mainly hydrogen and carbon dioxide gases. This causes all sorts of digestive symptoms including diarrhoea, abdominal pain, bloating and flatulence.

If you think you may be suffering from fructose intolerance, it might be worth asking your doctor about a test known as the hydrogen breath test. This detects abnormal levels of hydrogen from your breath, which usually indicates fructose intolerance. Bear in mind, however, that some of the symptoms described can be similar to those experienced by Candida sufferers due to the yeast feeding on sugars and giving off gases. If fructose intolerance is diagnosed, I advise you to consult a reputable nutritional therapist who will be able to devise an individual nutritional programme suited to your needs (see Useful Information, page 301).

Identifying problem foods

If you think you have a problem with any of the foods listed in this chapter, then I advise you to refer to Chapter 9 (page 187), where you will find important information on how to have yourself tested for food intolerances.

Food rotation

One of the best methods of relieving food intolerances is to introduce a food rotation diet. This approach works on the principle that you will have already had a food intolerance test, which has not only identified the foods that you should avoid but has also identified those you are less sensitive to and may eat on an infrequent basis, usually once every four days. Intolerance tests that involve analysing IgG antibody reactions (see also Chapter 3, page 15), such as the quantitative ELISA test (enzyme linked immunosorbent assay), conducted by the York Test Laboratories in the UK, are capable of measuring the degree of sensitivity to each food tested hence the description: quantitative. In effect, this means that you can still eat the foods that you have a slight sensitivity to, but only once every four days. By adopting this approach you avoid stressing your immune system because it's not constantly challenged by the food allergen, and your diet is therefore more varied. Having that variety is a good thing because if your diet is too narrow and you repeatedly eat the same things every day, you are more likely to become sensitive to those foods as well. Believe me, I speak from personal experience here: I once became intolerant to carrots and avocados simply because I was eating so many of them in an average week. Fortunately, in my case, after eliminating them from my diet for a few months, I was able to reintroduce both foods without any adverse effects.

Cross-reactions

When it comes to food rotation it's really important to bear in mind that foods are grouped in families so it's possible that if you're sensitive to, let's say, carrots, you might also have a problem with parsnips because they belong to the same family and cross-reactions may occur. Foods from any one family can be eaten on the same day, but not eaten again until the next three days have elapsed. The following example, which is based on someone whose test results indicate a slight sensitivity to crab, cucumber, apples and potatoes, will help to make this clearer.

Day 1	*Day 2*	*Day 3*	*Day 4*
Potato	Apple	Cucumber	Crab
Aubergine	Cider	Courgette	Crayfish
Tomato	Pear	Honeydew melon	Lobster
Sesame	Rosehip	Pumpkin	Shrimp
Tahini	Crab apple	Squash	Prawn

When considering the above example, bear in mind that you can also eat the everyday foods that you know you're not intolerant to. The rotation just means that you can choose any of the foods listed from the same family on any one of the four days then leave a gap of three days before having any of the foods from that group again.

Re-introducing foods

The question I am most frequently asked is: 'Will I ever be able to re-introduce wheat (or whatever it happens to be) back into my diet?' This very much depends on the individual but there is a protocol that I use to gauge whether a food can be safely re-introduced into the diet. Here's how it works...

After excluding the offending food for three months, try eating a little of it again. If no adverse reaction is noted during the following three days, try eating that food again. Again, if no adverse reaction occurs, you should be able to eat that food in moderation. The three-day gap allows for any delayed reactions to show up. If you want to test yourself for another food, follow the same protocol and observe the results. Remember to leave the three-day gap before trying that food again.

The reason why it's sometimes possible to re-introduce foods after excluding them from your diet altogether for three months is because your immune system can 'forget' that the specific food allergen is an enemy and will not react to that food in the the way that it used to. I hasten to point out, however, that this doesn't happen in cases of true allergy such as coeliac disease when the individual sufferer must avoid gluten for life.

IMPORTANT

When re-introducing a food, choose only the purest form available. For example, when trying wheat after the required period of abstinence, opt for a wheat product made from 100% wheat otherwise other items in the equation could cloud the issue. For example, some people make the mistake of eating a slice of bread and because this is likely to contain yeast and possibly other ingredients such as preservatives, then the result cannot rule out that you're not reacting to those things. Similarly, when testing yourself for cow's dairy produce, opt for something like plain yoghurt, preferably organic. If you get no reaction over the three days, then try another dairy product such as milk. Eggs should be separated into yolk and white because you could be reacting to either of them. Again, I advise you to choose organic because there is less chance of any additives such as hormones distorting the result.

9

Identifying your food intolerances: tests that work

As I've already stated in Chapter 3 (see page 15), strictly speaking, food allergies are very different to food intolerances. Those who suspect they may have a sensitivity to a particular food (or foods) will usually visit their doctor in the hope that he will refer them to a specialist who will conduct the appropriate tests to identify the problem. Typically, this will involve the following scenario:

- You visit your doctor to explain that you suspect that you are reacting adversely to a food (or foods).
- He refers you to a specialist who deals with testing for food allergies.
- You are given a skin pin-prick test which is designed to identify IgE antibody reactions to a specific range of commonly eaten foods – for example, wheat, dairy and nuts.
- You await the results of the tests which are sent to your doctor.
- The results may or may not be conclusive. For example, you might be convinced that you have a problem with

wheat because every time you eat pasta you feel bloated and drowsy. However, the test suggests your suspicions are unfounded.

- You feel frustrated and confused because you strongly suspect that certain foods affect you but the test results indicate the opposite.

Perhaps you've already experienced this type of scenario, in which case you'll definitely identify with those feelings of frustration and confusion. So why haven't the tests identified your problem? Simply because this type of test looks at IgE immune reactions and not IgG reactions normally associated with food intolerances. This is also the case when someone is suspected of suffering from a gluten allergy, otherwise known as coeliac disease. Suspected sufferers have their blood tested for antibodies to gluten. Sometimes the blood tests fail to identify a problem even though the person being tested is absolutely convinced that they react badly to grains containing gluten (these grains include wheat, barley, oats and rye). In actual fact the test has very likely produced accurate results. In other words, they have indicated quite rightly that you don't have an allergy to gluten. However, this is the crux of the problem because you may instead have an intolerance and this state is becoming more widely recognised by doctors. In fact, a very well known doctor in the UK was speaking on national television recently about gluten allergy. I was interested to hear him acknowledge that there can be different degrees of gluten sensitivity. In my experience this is very true and usually applies to people who have delayed reactions to gluten and not the instant reactions associated with a true gluten allergy, which is evident in coeliac disease.

Choosing the best test for you

Unfortunately, since testing for IgG type allergies/intolerances is not always offered to patients (and certainly not on the UK's National Health Service), it is up to the individual to seek out a reputable company to carry out reliable tests. In addition, it is possible to carry out some simple testing on oneself at home. To help simplify this matter of choice, I have included here an explanation of what I consider to be the best testing methods currently available.

The Pulse Test

The idea behind this approach is to avoid all foods that you suspect for a period of fourteen days. You then have to re-introduce each one at a time, leaving a forty-eight hour gap in between each food being tested. The procedure is as follows:

- While sitting down, take your resting pulse rate prior to eating the food you are testing.
- After eating the food, take your pulse rate after ten minutes, then thirty minutes and finally, sixty minutes.
- If there is a significant increase in your pulse rate of higher than ten points or you become aware of any adverse reactions, avoid that food for twenty-four hours before testing the next one.

Advantages: This method does not involve you in any financial cost. It is a fairly accurate method of isolating the foods that you are sensitive to.

Disadvantages: Some symptoms may not manifest themselves for several hours or even days later. Leaving out certain foods may only result in slight, less discernible changes. The procedure requires discipline and patience to monitor the results effectively.

Electro-Dermal Testing

In the early 1950s German doctor Reinhold Voll developed an electronic testing device that could locate acupuncture points on the body electrically. Not only was he successful in finding those acupuncture points (which have been known to Chinese acupuncturists for thousands of years), he also demonstrated that they had a different resistance to a minute electrical current passed through the body compared to the adjacent tissues. Significantly, a number of other researchers have verified his findings, concluding that electrical conductance at the acupuncture points is measurably greater than the surrounding tissue.

Voll then proceeded to identify correlations between disease states and changes in electrical resistance of the various acupuncture points. He believed that if he could identify electrical changes in specific acupuncture points associated with certain diseases, then it might be possible to detect those diseases more easily or even sooner, thus providing the opportunity for earlier medical intervention. To this end he was very successful because he managed to identify many acupuncture points relating to specific conditions. For example, he found that people suffering from lung cancer had abnormal readings on the acupuncture points referred to by Chinese physicians as 'lung points'. This kind of technology can also be used for allergy testing and studies continue to show it to be as accurate as, or more accurate than other forms of allergy testing. For example, an allergy study[1] of six diagnostic measures was conducted by four doctors: Julia J. Tsuei, M.D., Carl W.

1 Tseui, J., Lehman, C., Fred, M.K., Lam, F. and Zhu, D. A 'Food Allergy study utilizing the EAV Technique', Amer. J. Acupuncture, vol. 12, No. 2, 1984; 105–16.

Lehman, M.D., Fred M.K. Lam Jr., M.D. and David A.H. Zhu, M.D. The techniques were performed on 30 volunteers. Five of these techniques are widely recognised procedures for allergy testing: namely, history and food challenge, skin, RAST (radioallergosorbent test; a blood test used to investigate food sensitivities) and IgE tests. The sixth method of testing was based upon electro-acupuncture (EAV). Results showed a high degree of compatibility with the other five tests, particularly the food challenge test, which is often regarded as one of the most reliable methods of determining food sensitivity.

Personally, I have worked with this kind of testing for a number of years now and I have found it to be an accurate method of identifying food intolerances. For more information, refer to Useful Information, page xx at the end of this book.

Advantages: This type of testing can identify food intolerances, which are usually more difficult to detect than food allergies because the former may result in a delayed reaction to a food (or foods). The test doesn't require a blood sample and the results of each item being tested are instantaneous. With the latest technology, the person being tested can see their results on a computer screen. In addition to this, they are given a printout of the results.

Disadvantages: Inconsistent results may ensue if the person conducting the testing is not proficient in using the machine.

IgG Food Intolerance Testing

This form of testing is based on the analysis of a blood sample that is sent to a laboratory, where a procedure known as a quantitative IgG ELISA test is carried out. The blood sample is tested for IgG reactions to a wide range of foods and the quantitative element of the procedure means that the test shows not only if you're sensitive to a specific food, but the level of that sensitivity. Obviously, all the foods that you strongly react to must be eliminated from your diet. However, the foods you are less sensitive to can be eaten on a rotation basis, as explained in Chapter 8 (see page 184).

One company that carries out this form of testing based in the UK is Yorktest. The Yorktest foodSCAN tests are reputed to be the first and only scientifically proven IgG tests, having been assessed in October 2004 in a double-blind placebo controlled clinical trial designed by the University Hospital of South Manchester and a prospective audit on food intolerance and its effects on migraines. This test is now available to the public as a home test kit. A small sample of blood is taken using a simple pinprick. Once complete, you send the sample to the laboratory where it is analysed, following which the results are sent to you in the post. See also Useful Information, page 301.

Advantages: An indication of the level of sensitivity to specific foods is useful as foods that you are mildly sensitive to can still be included in your diet on a rotation basis. A wide range of foods is usually included in the test and provided the tests are carried out by a reputable company the results are deemed to be accurate. Some companies such as YORKTEST (www.yorktest.com) provide follow-up advice from their qualified nutritionists based on your test results.

Disadvantages: Inaccurate results may occur when testing is carried out by companies without a proven track record.

Part II

10

What causes food intolerances?

O ver the years, many clients have asked me if food allergies and intolerances are on the increase. It's difficult to be precise, however all I can say is that I continue to see an increasing number of people who test positive for food intolerances and more often than not their health improves significantly after eliminating the offending foods. Certainly, the general consensus among natural therapists and many nutritionists is that allergies per se are on the increase and symptomatic of our modern way of eating and living.

So what is it about our twenty-first century lifestyle that predisposes us towards the development of allergies and food intolerances? I believe that the so-called Western diet, which is based on a high intake of refined carbohydrates such as white flour products and sugars, salt, saturated fats, processed foods and chemical additives has played a significant role in bringing about many diseases including obesity, allergies and intolerances. This is in stark contrast to our prehistoric ancestors, who existed on a much more natural diet consisting of fruits, vegetables, nuts, seeds and, depending on geographical location, some meats and fish. Furthermore, our stone-age ancestors ate only organically grown food and this, of course, was devoid of toxic pesticides, fungicides and artificial nitrates. Their diet would have provided them with an abundance of vitamins, minerals and other nutrients. Instead of eating too many artery-clogging fats, additives and salt, they consumed lots of healthy fats (mostly from plants), low sodium and no chemical additives. The question is, does this way of eating have a positive influence on health? The following true story may give us some vital clues.

The tale of the people of Hunza

Hunza is a state that is situated in the extreme northernmost point of India. For many years the people who lived in this remote, and then inaccessible region were renowned for their impressive longevity and good health. The late Sir Robert McCarrison, a pioneer of nutritional research, lived among them for a number of years. During this time he observed that their diet consisted of unrefined wheat, barley, maize, vegetables and an abundance of apricots dried in the sun that formed a large part of their diet. In studying the health of the Hunza people, Sir Robert observed their diet was very pure and although they lived a very frugal existence, they suffered from virtually none of the diseases so prevalent in modern society. Cancer was rare, as was diabetes; also strokes, obesity and heart disease.

What eventually happened to these people should be a lesson to us all: with the advent of civilisation came better access to this remote and mountainous region. This led to imports of processed foods such as white sugar, white flour and alcohol.

Unfortunately their once pure and natural diet became corrupted by all this and for the first time in their history they began to suffer from the so-called chronic diseases that appear to be so accepted by our modern society. If ever a lesson from the past should be heeded, then this surely must be it. In fact, the message could not be more emphatic: We were meant to live on natural foods designed by nature to provide us with all the elements we need to sustain good health! We were not designed to live on unnatural processed foods such as those made from white flour, refined sugar, unhealthy fats, high in salt and laced with additives. If we ignore these natural laws, we become significantly more vulnerable to chronic disease including allergies and obesity.

The important thing here is that by living on a natural diet not only do we supply the body with all the nutrients it needs to maintain optimum health, we also minimise the degree of toxins our cells have to deal with on a day-to-day basis. This is our greatest defence against disease and it is a view postulated by many of the world's leading natural health gurus for many years, including Swiss naturopath and herbalist, Dr Alfred Vogel, and Professor Arnold Ehret. Ehret was an expert on the use of fasting and fruit diets for curing disease. He not only cured himself of Bright's Disease (a kidney disease) using these methods, but went on to help many people heal themselves of numerous serious illnesses. The view of how toxicity and nutrient deficiencies can result in the manifestation of disease in the body is also consistent with the opinions of Raymond Francis, internationally recognised expert on optimal health and author of the ground-breaking book, *Never Be Sick Again* (see also page 302). Francis, a former biochemist, was gravely ill in hospital but he saved his own life with a nutritional approach. This extract from his book illustrates his view of how nutritional deficiencies and toxins can affect the body on a cellular level:

> Cells malfunction only if they suffer from a lack of nutrients (deficiency), toxic damage (toxicity) or a combination of both. Preventing these two causes of disease is made possible by our ability to choose how we live our lives. Health depends on the choices we make.

Furthermore, he postulates that obesity is the direct result of cells that have been deprived of nutrients, this being the consequence of living on a diet that comprises nutrient deficient processed foods. Francis reasons that when this happens the body feels compelled to eat more. Or, as he puts it: 'A body that is starving of nutrients seeks out more food, and weight gain likely results.'

The High Allergenic Diet

In addition to high toxicity and lack of important nutrients, could it be that our modern diet is too heavily weighted in favour of foods known to be highly allergenic? When the most frequently eaten foods in Westernised countries are analysed, the only conclusion can be that the most commonly consumed foods are based around wheat, dairy products, sugar and foods containing yeast. As I have already stated (see page 180), constant frequent exposure to foods such as wheat may be strongly implicated in the escalation of wheat and gluten allergies and intolerances. Also, don't forget that grains have only featured in the human diet for around 10,000 years – a very short time in evolutionary terms and certainly not long enough for the human species to have adapted to eating such foods.

Dr. Doug Graham, author of the book, *Grain Damage*, also subscribes to the view that grains are not a natural part of our diet. In another of his books, *On Nutrition and Physical Performance: A Handbook for Athletes and Fitness Enthusiasts* (see also page 302), he has this to say about grain consumption: 'There is no model in nature for human grain consumption. Our anthropoid primate cousins like the chimpanzees, gorillas, orang-utans and mandrills consume no grains. All animals, with the exception of humans and their domesticated animals, consume only the foods to which they are biologically adapted. And none of them, with the exception of a few varieties of birds and insects, consume grains.'

Personally, I feel this is a very convincing argument and one consistent with what we know about the high allergenic properties of grains. Other factors likely to increase your chances of developing food allergies and intolerances include:

- Over-use of antibiotics
- The early introduction of cow's milk in infancy
- Increased use of NSAIDS (Non-Steroidal Anti-Inflammatory Drugs)
- Leaky gut syndrome
- Dysbiosis – an imbalance of gut bacteria
- Hereditary influence – an inherited predisposition towards the development of allergies/intolerances
- Food additives
- Toxins

Gut bacteria: How the balance becomes disturbed

As already discussed in Chapter 7 on the subject of Candida (see page 135), the intestines are home to billions of bacteria, both friendly and unfriendly. The total weight of all these bacteria amounts to an incredible 1 kilo (2lb) – or put it another way, the equivalent of a bag of sugar. As long as the intestines are well populated with the friendly bacteria, unfriendly strains cannot cause any problems. However, as you'll now be aware, should the balance shift in favour of the unfriendly bacteria and other potentially pathogenic organisms, such as yeasts then the end result can be digestive dysfunction. When this happens, the permeability of the intestines can increase, resulting in larger food particles passing through the intestine walls and entering the bloodstream. These foreign particles can trigger off allergies and intolerances. Therefore, an imbalance of the gut flora (sometimes referred to as dysbiosis) can be a chief culprit in increasing the allergic potential of the individual.

As I've already elaborated on, unfortunately our modern style of living as well as the increasing use of various drugs can adversely upset the balance of these healthy bacteria. If we take into account the influence of the foregoing factors on the lining of the digestive tract in addition to the effects of an unhealthy diet, we have the recipe for the development of food allergies and intolerances.

11

How food intolerances can zap your energy and sabotage your efforts to lose weight

Do any of these conditions apply to you?
- Feeling tired most of the time
- Lacking the drive and enthusiasm to do things
- Drowsiness
- Feeling moody or depressed
- An inability to lose weight.

If you have experienced one or more of these conditions, especially if they are persistent, then the underlying cause could be food intolerance. Of course, it's true that all of these conditions are very common, especially given the hectic pace of modern life and we are also subjected to many stresses including poor diet, exposure to numerous pollutants and demands on our time and energy. All, or any of these factors can result in the depletion of the body's energy levels, ultimately resulting in any of the above conditions. This is the very reason why so many of us rely on stimulants to help keep us going. Stimulants such as caffeine and sugars may give us a brief boost in energy only to deplete us of that same energy in the long run. Having said this, I have lost count of the number of food intolerance sufferers who have said to me, 'I am so lacking in energy all the time!' Or 'I feel so tired, bloated and overweight!' The fact is that while the foregoing conditions are not always understood by doctors to be symptomatic of a food allergy or intolerance, they are widely recognised by many natural health practitioners, including many nutritionists.

You may well ask, what is happening to the food intolerance sufferer that results in the manifestation of such debilitating conditions in the first place? In fact, I have asked myself the same question many times over the years and my research and experience has led me to conclude that while food allergies and intolerances are often a major influence in terms of weight loss issues, there are a number of inter-related factors, singly or collectively, that block your attempts to lose weight and often result in you gaining weight in the first place.

How food intolerance can stress the immune system

Consider this: each time the immune system reacts to a certain food it calls on the body's resources to deal with it. This means galvanising the body's defences in the shape of immune cells sent to apprehend the perceived 'invader'. If this happens ten times a day, then the immune system reacts ten times – it's as simple as that! The trouble is that all this activity requires energy. The more the immune system is stressed by being challenged by the allergen, the greater the amount of energy and resources used up. To further compound the problem, every time a food evokes an immune response then the immune system uses up vital supplies of vitamins and minerals. No wonder people with food allergies and intolerances are always tired!

Food intolerance and malabsorption

From reading the first part of this book, you will already be aware that food intolerances damage the lining of the digestive system. The resulting inflammation can lead to many of the most common symptoms associated with food intolerances. Moreover, this damage can also lead to the poor absorption of nutrients through the lining of the small intestine. The end result can be a deficiency in several key vitamins and minerals. When it comes to energy levels, this may be highly significant because the body needs these nutrients to convert energy in the cells. The overall effect on the body can be a significant lack of energy.

The energy nutrients

Key nutrients needed to convert fuel from food into energy in the body's cells include: B1, B2, B3 and B5, vitamin C, iron, copper and Co-enzyme Q10. In addition, copper, magnesium and iron minerals are needed. Some nutrients such as chromium, known as the Glucose Tolerance Factor (GTF), are required to regulate the hormones that control blood sugar levels. This is vital in terms of keeping energy levels in the body stable and also in weight control. Equally important, a deficiency of iron and the vitamins B6, B12 and folic acid can lead to low energy levels because these nutrients are involved in red blood cell formation – red blood cells are needed to transport oxygen (used for energy) around the body. Those suffering from food intolerances are often deficient in many of these nutrients and so again, it's hardly surprising they become tired and lethargic.

Toxins

Another name for toxins is poisons. Everyone has a certain level of toxins stored in their body – naturopaths and nutritional therapists sometimes refer to this as an individual's 'toxic load'. We are more likely to have a higher level of toxins if we eat too many processed foods and choose unhealthy lifestyle habits such as smoking and/or drinking too much alcohol. Toxins can interfere with normal function of our cells, which in turn interferes with normal energy production in the body. This internal cellular pollution also uses up key nutrients and may result in weight gain.

How food intolerance can cause digestive imbalance

There is another important observation that I have made over the years: namely, that food intolerance not only causes damage to the lining of the digestive system, it also creates disruption of major digestive components such as a depletion in the hydrochloric acid level in the stomach and a low level of digestive enzymes and gut flora. How did I know this was linked to the presence of food intolerance? Quite simply, because once the individual concerned began to exclude the offending food (or foods) from his/her diet, a re-test several months later nearly always indicated that the digestive components had gradually returned to normal levels. This proved to both the client and myself that by eliminating the offending food, the body was able to heal itself in terms of repairing the gut lining and also by restoring normal levels of digestive components. I soon concluded that this was a major factor in determining why it was that a previously overweight individual would begin to lose weight. In other words, if the digestive system is working better, then food is digested more efficiently, resulting in weight loss.

Food addiction

As explained in Chapter 2, it's not unusual for a person to be addicted to the very foods they're sensitive to. Remember, temporarily eating the very foods to which you're intolerant can actually make you feel better. When the effects wear off you tend to crave the same foods and so it goes on. This is why, for instance, a wheat-sensitive person will often crave bread, biscuits and pretty much anything made from wheat.

As discussed earlier, it's also thought that food addiction can affect the brain chemistry because endorphin-like substances are produced when you eat certain foods. These make us feel good but again, when their effects wear off, we crave more of them. High-allergenic foods such as wheat and dairy produce are two of the biggest culprits. Such food addiction can result in binge eating, thus perpetuating the feel-good factor, which in turn predisposes the food addict to obesity.

Candidiasis

As discussed in Chapter 7, candidiasis, or yeast overgrowth, can seriously disrupt the digestive system, producing toxins that overload the liver and present a constant challenge to the immune system. All of these factors may result in weight regulation problems. Candida sufferers who embark upon an anti-Candida programme frequently report a significant weight loss, especially in the first few weeks.

Low energy and the exercise factor

It stands to reason that if your energy is depleted by any or all of the foregoing factors, you're not going to want to exercise. This may be a serious disadvantage to the person who wishes to lose weight because exercise can be a major influence when it comes to burning up excess calories and speeding up your metabolism. It's true that if you manage to identify and eradicate your food intolerances as well as adhere to a healthy diet, then the chances are you're going to lose both fluid and fat. However, if you incorporate regular aerobic exercise into your life, you will undoubtedly accelerate your loss of weight. Identifying and eradicating your intolerances often leads to an improvement in your energy levels. When this happens you will almost certainly feel more like exercising, even if it's just a brisk walk every day.

The factors that deplete your energy and result in weight gain

Depleted immune system Junk food diet Malabsorption of nutrients	WEIGHT
Deficiency of key nutrients needed for energy production and maintenance of the immune system	GAIN
Digestive imbalance Food Addiction/Cravings	LOW
Candidiasis Lack of exercise Water retention Toxins	ENERGY

The solution to low energy and weight regulation problems

Naturopaths and most nutritional therapists maintain that to overcome a disease state within the body you have to reverse the process that eventually led to that disease manifesting itself in the first place. In other words, if you create the right conditions then the body is often capable of healing itself.

When it comes to increasing one's energy levels and losing excess weight, this same principal applies. So, in terms of food intolerances, we obviously need to identify them and then eliminate the offending foods from our diet. However, it is also vital that we adhere to a healthy diet and lifestyle. What's the point in eliminating the foods that trigger off problems with your health and weight, only to continue with a junk food diet and unhealthy lifestyle? Remember, it may have been these very conditions that caused your food intolerances and weight gain in the first place!

The remaining chapters in this book address the key factors that can influence your overall health and wellbeing. By the judicious application of the advice that follows, not only will you increase your resistance to food intolerance, but also set in place the conditions your body needs to achieve true health and improved long-term weight regulation.

12

Healthy eating: the key to long-term weight control

Your digestive system will thank you for choosing to eat mostly natural foods by reducing any propensity to develop further intolerances. And it's not only your digestive system that will benefit for your immune system is the key to how you react to all substances that enter the body whether through food and drink or via the skin or airways. If your immune system isn't compromised by internal pollution and deficiencies of vital nutrients, you're far less likely to develop new intolerances and your ability to overcome current intolerances is enhanced. Furthermore, by paying attention to your diet and lifestyle in this way, you are much more likely not only to shed those excess pounds but to keep them off too! Study the key components of a healthy diet below.

The importance of fresh fruit and vegetables

Remember that every time you eat fresh fruit and vegetables, especially in their raw state, you supply yourself with a cocktail of vitamins, minerals, antioxidants, amino acids, enzymes and a whole variety of phytochemicals that work together synergistically to bring about good health. Phytochemicals are natural chemicals from edible plants that are good for our health. Tomatoes contain lycopene, for example, which is thought to exert a protective effect against certain cancers. This is why, ideally, the bulk of your diet should consist of fruit and vegetables with at least 50% in their raw state. It's worth remembering that raw foods contain enzymes and other natural compounds that are destroyed by heat. Therefore, although some cooked vegetables can be nutritious when cooked with minimal heat, generally speaking they are inferior to raw foods.

Daily eating plan

- Include at least one salad a day as part of a meal or on its own.
- Eat at least 3–4 pieces of fruit per day. If you don't enjoy many fruits and you are not following an anti-Candida diet, try making freshly made smoothies. If you are following an anti-Candida diet then avoid smoothies because their high sugar content will exacerbate your condition.
- Include a variety of multi-coloured foods such as red peppers, beetroot, squashes and carrots in your diet. These are rich in health promoting and protective phytochemicals. Broccoli, watercress, sweet potatoes and sprouted seeds such as alfalfa sprouts are all rich in health-promoting and protective antioxidants.
- When cooking, try to steam foods as much as possible or lightly stir-fry.
- Eat as many whole foods as possible and minimise your consumption of processed and refined foods.
- Buy organic foods where possible. If using commercially grown fruit and vegetables, peel skins and discard outer

leaves; wash thoroughly. Normal rinsing in water will only remove some of the pesticide residues on commercially grown fruit and vegetables, but you can wash them in a mixture of 3 tablespoons vinegar and 45ml/3 tbsp/4 cups water. This will help to remove pesticides.

- With the exception of those following an anti-Candida diet, include some fermented foods such as live yoghurt, miso (seaweed) and sauerkraut in your diet.

- Take a good multivitamin/mineral supplement daily (see Useful Information, page 303).

- Use only pure filtered or spring water for drinking purposes.

- Include the whole grains that you are not intolerant to (e.g. if you are not intolerant to rice, choose the wholegrain variety rather than white rice which has been refined).

- If meat is included in your diet, select mostly white meats such as chicken (preferably free-range organic). Avoid cured and processed meats such as corned beef, ham and bacon as these foods contain chemical additives and are high in salt.

- Include some oily fish such as wild salmon or mackerel two or three times per week.

Opt for organic foods

When I was a young man living in Sunderland, north-east England, organic food was a rarity, not being generally available in supermarkets and local shops. If you wanted organic fruit and vegetables you had to find an organic farm or a health food shop specialising in that sort of thing. Mind you, that didn't stop me from paying regular visits to local allotments where some of the growers were not great fans of poisoning their produce with chemical sprays, etc. Admittedly, they had to find natural ways of controlling pests but the end result was food that not only looked mouthwateringly scrumptious but tasted as good as it looked – all this, and the added bonus of being pesticide-free!

Those early forays into the world of organic produce took place in the 1970s. At the time I could never have envisaged how things would change in just a few decades. These days we can walk into just about any supermarket and purchase a wide range of organic fruits, vegetables, meats, dairy produce, nuts, seeds, cereals, pulses, honey, bread and a whole lot more! What's more, if we get involved in an organic box scheme, we can even have fresh organic produce delivered straight to our door.

Without doubt, organic food is one of the fastest growing industries in many countries around the world. Of course the reason for this is that people are becoming increasingly worried about the chemicals used in agriculture. Many parents are particularly concerned about the amount of chemicals found in everyday foods such as fruit, vegetables and dairy products that their children ingest. This situation has been highlighted in random tests on produce such as leafy vegetables, carrots, apples and strawberries and often reveals levels of pesticides that are above the recommended safe levels.

Safety assessments

In safety assessments for pesticides, each chemical is looked at in isolation, however there is a basic flaw when using this approach, namely the fact that most commercially grown produce contains not one but often a mixture of pesticide residues. This was highlighted in the year 2000 in the Annual Report of the Pesticide Residues Committee, an organization which monitors levels of pesticide residues in UK produce (see Useful Information, p304) which revealed one third of the apples and nearly half of the pears tested contained residues of more than one pesticide.

Very little research has been conducted into the safety of pesticides. However, some studies have indicated that these chemical cocktails may be detrimental to the immune system; also carcinogenic and could potentially affect behaviour. Some pesticides commonly found in our food have been identified by the European Union as possible hormone disruptors. This happens because the chemicals actually mimic the body's natural hormones or block them from working normally. Hormone disruptors are thought to be linked with falling sperm counts as well as earlier than normal puberty among girls. Nevertheless, whatever conclusions we might come to from these studies, to my mind there is one overriding factor: namely this, that there is not one so-called expert anywhere in the world who can categorically state that pesticides do not cause damage to humans!

Of course, when presented with the facts, very few people are happy with the idea that they are being exposed to chemicals that have the potential to cause harm. This is why an increasing number opt for organic produce whenever possible. Part of the problem is that the majority of us are insulated from the business end of the food-growing process. If you were able to see farmers spraying their crops with potentially harmful chemical cocktails, ask yourself whether you would still be happy to go out and purchase commercially grown fruit, vegetables and grains to feed yourself or your children.

Cost implications

Yes, it's true that organic produce is more expensive and this can be a serious setback for people who want to buy more organic food but find it cost-prohibitive. This is especially true of parents with large families, of course. However, if you find yourself in this kind of situation, it might still be possible for you to make some changes and this is better than basing your diet solely on produce that has been grown using conventional methods Also, when it comes to choice, you may be able to prioritise: in other words, try to avoid the most heavily sprayed crops such as strawberries, apples and green leafy vegetables such as lettuce. The highest usage of pesticide is found in commercially grown strawberries and these sometimes contain as many as thirty different pesticide residues. If you think I may be exaggerating, consider this: strawberries are often used as a reference standard which gives us a basis for comparison when evaluating the pesticides found in crops. They are given a score of 100 and other produce has a score relative to that. Here is a general guide that you can use when deciding which commercially grown fruits and vegetables to omit from your shopping list:

100 points	**Strawberries**
50 points or more	**Berries such as blackberries, raspberries, cherries, apricots, nectarines and pears**
28 points	**Potatoes**
19 points	**Bananas**
18 points	**Carrots**
16 points	**Green peas**
15 points and under	**Broccoli, Brussels sprouts, cauliflower**
5–10 points	**Onions, corn and spring onions**
4 points	**Avocados**

Nutritional value

Another good reason to opt for organic produce whenever possible is commercially grown crops have been shown to be lower in the important vitamins and minerals that are especially important for young growing children. This is because the soil in which the crops are grown is depleted in minerals due to the heavy use of artificial nitrates. Compare this to organic farming, where natural fertilisers and crop rotation are used to replenish the goodness in the soil.

Good reasons to go organic...

- Organic food is nutritious
- It's also safe
- Organic food is produced from GM-free ingredients
- The employment of organic farming methods usually means the farm animals are well looked after
- Organic husbandry methods result in far less risk of developing mad-cow disease (BSE) as a result of eating infected beef
- Organic food production helps safeguard the environment and the plants and animals living in that environment
- It simply tastes better!
- Organic food uses a sustainable form of agriculture because goodness is put back into the soil
- Finally... it is free from harmful chemical residues that may damage your digestive tract and increase your allergic potential.

13

Healthy fats:
their role in helping you
to lose weight

If you want to speed up your metabolism and reduce the likelihood of succumbing to arthritis, heart disease, hardening of the arteries, low energy, eczema, poor concentration, problems associated with the immune system, cancer and hyperactivity, eat fat. FAT IS GOOD FOR YOU! But before you come to the conclusion that I have well and truly lost the plot, I hasten to point out that I'm talking here about *good* fats, otherwise known as essential fats that cannot be made by the body. Such fats have to come from the foods we eat. Of course we all know that certain fats, eaten to excess, can be very harmful to our health. I'm referring here to saturated fats, which are found in milk, cheese and meats, among others. We also have refined fats known as trans-fatty acids found in such products as mass-produced chocolate, most margarine and some packaged foods.

Basically most people brought up on a typical Western diet eat too many saturated fats and not enough healthy fats. Saturated fats are implicated as a major causative factor in the development of heart disease, thrombosis, hardening of the arteries, high levels of bad cholesterol, obesity and other degenerative illnesses.

Types of fat

The three most important types of fat are: saturated fat, polyunsaturated fat and monounsaturated fat. All fats are made from fatty acids and these are created from a chain of carbon atoms, to which hydrogen atoms are attached. Imagine a caterpillar shape with 'arms' sticking out horizontally: each 'arm' has the potential to have a hydrogen atom attached to it. Fats are classified according to how 'saturated' they are. Saturation simply refers to the number of hydrogen atoms attached to the molecules of fat.

So, what is saturated fat?

Where saturated fat is concerned, each fat molecule is covered with hydrogen atoms (all the 'arms' are full). In other words, it is completely saturated. As already stated, this type of fat is known to increase the risk of chronic health conditions, particularly those associated with the cardiovascular system. Saturated fats are easily distinguishable from other fats because they remain solid at room temperature (butter, for example). They are mostly found in foods from animal sources but they also occur in some plant foods, sometimes referred to as tropical fats (for example, coconut oil).

Saturated fats found in foods

- Coconut oil
- Coconut
- Palm oil
- Palm kernel oil
- Cocoa butter
- Butter
- Low-fat cheese
- Chocolate

- Lard
- Beef
- Chicken
- Turkey

- Hydrogenated fat
- Milk cream
- Whole milk
- Cheeses

So, what is polyunsaturated fat?

These fats are not saturated with hydrogen atoms; that is to say, there are a number of sites around each fat molecule where hydrogen atoms could be attached. For this reason, they are very unstable and quickly damaged when subjected to heat, as in frying and also when exposed to light and air. Nevertheless, polyunsaturated fats, when extracted properly and also when protected from air, light and heat, can be good for our health. The most well known of these are the Omega 3 and Omega 6 polyunsaturated fatty acids, which have a lot of important functions in the body. They are very influential in terms of brain function, lowering LDL (bad) cholesterol and in reducing inflammation. Children who have been given supplements containing these fatty acids have exhibited significant improvements in behaviour, attention span and even cognitive ability. Unlike saturated fats, they are liquid at room temperature.

Polyunsaturated fats found in foods

- Safflower oil
- Sunflower oil
- Soybean oil
- Rapeseed oil
- Corn oil
- Walnut oil
- Sesame oil
- Soybeans

- Tofu
- Margarine
- Salad dressings
- Nuts
- Seeds

So, what is monounsaturated fat?

Monounsaturated fats are also not saturated and as the name suggests, each fat molecule has just one space for one hydrogen atom. An increasing number of experts are of the opinion that monounsaturated fats are good for us and may help to ward off heart disease. Olive oil is largely composed of monounsaturated fats and is consumed in significant amounts in the so-called Mediterranean Diet, an eating plan thought to reduce the incidence of cardiovascular disease and some cancers.

Unlike polyunsaturated oils such as sunflower, olive oil is the one that is considered to be acceptable for cooking purposes (e.g. stir-frying). This is because monounsaturated fats, due to their partial saturation with hydrogen atoms, are much more stable when heated and less likely to form harmful substances. It is best to use extra virgin olive oil for this purpose though as the other types are refined. Coconut butter is an alternative to olive oil. Unlike saturated fats from ordinary butter and meats, which contain long-chain saturated fat, coconut butter has only short-chain saturated fat, which is not associated with health problems such as an increased risk of heart disease.

Monounsaturated fat found in foods

- Olive oil
- Coconut oil
- Olives
- Canola oil
- Canola seeds
- Avocado oil
- Avocados
- Peanut oil
- Peanuts
- Peanut butter
- Cashew nuts

So, what are trans-fatty acids?

These fats occur as a result of a chemical process called hydrogenation. This involves exposing unsaturated fats such as sunflower oil to hydrogen gas, which then makes the fats more saturated and therefore more solid at room temperature. Ever wondered why chocolate and margarine stay solid at room temperature? Have a look at the ingredients and you'll see that most of these products contain hydrogenated fats.

Trans-fats tend to elevate LDL (bad) cholesterol. The cells of the human body require essential fatty acids to function properly but unfortunately, trans-fats interfere with their absorption. Children these days often eat a lot of foods containing hydrogenated fats so unless your kids are unusual in this respect, their absorption of the healthy fats will be compromised.

Polyunsaturated fats and the two most important fatty acids

Omega 3 and Omega 6, the two most important fatty acids, are contained in polyunsaturated fats. These are the good guys! Both are converted into hormone-like substances known as prostaglandins, which have lots of important functions within the body. Unfortunately, most people, including children, are deficient in both Omega 3 and Omega 6 fats because they don't eat enough of the foods containing them. Having said that, the majority of people tend to be more deficient in Omega 3. This is hardly surprising when you consider that such ingredients as margarine and cooking oils (except olive oil) are high in Omega 6 fats. Moreover, as already stated, saturated and trans-fatty acids stop the body from effectively using good fats.

How Omega 3 fats can help you lose weight

Remember, these fats are essential for our health since the body cannot manufacture them. For this reason they are described as essential fatty acids. Omega 3 fats are found in abundance in flaxseed oil (otherwise known as linseed oil), hemp oil and rapeseed. As long as you consume fish oils or Omega 3- and 6-rich plant oils in your diet, you can be sure that you are getting enough of the essential fatty acids that are so important for your health. You can also sprinkle ground-up flaxseed onto breakfast cereals such as muesli, or onto salads or yoghurt.

Anti-inflammatory effects

The body converts Omega 3 fatty acids into hormone-like substances known as prostaglandin series three. These have anti-inflammatory effects and that is why they can be helpful in reducing the impact of allergies and intolerances. Most overweight people find it difficult to grasp the idea that Omega 3 fats can actually help us lose weight. This is because many of us have become 'fat phobic' and think in terms of all fats being bad for us. This is most definitely not the case because Omega 3 fats can help us to lose excess weight in the following ways:

- They actually *increase* the metabolic rate. This means that more fat and glucose are burned up in the body.
- Omega 3 fats help to make hormone-like substances in the body known as series three prostaglandins, which in turn can help the kidneys to expel excess water held in the tissues.
- They help to increase energy levels, resulting in a greater inclination to exercise which in turn helps to burn more calories.

Omega 6 fats

The most important component of the Omega 6 family is linoleic acid, which is converted by the body into gamma-linolenic acid (GLA). Two very rich sources of GLA are borage oil and evening primrose oil. Eventually the body converts GLA into the prostaglandin series one, a hormone-like substance which helps to prevent blood clots, decreases inflammation and helps insulin to work. This is good for weight regulation as it influences blood sugar levels.

The benefits of Omega 6 fats

- Blood is kept thin, thus preventing clots and obstructions
- Omega 6 fats relax blood vessels and help to keep them pliable
- Blood pressure is lowered
- Inflammation and pain is decreased
- Omega 6 fats help to maintain the water balance in the body
- They also improve nerve and immune function
- Omega 6 fats help insulin to work.

Getting the balance right

The ideal source of essential fatty acids should provide high levels of both Omega 3 and Omega 6. There is some debate about how much we should consume through our everyday diet. If the diet of our primitive hunter-gatherer ancestors is anything to go by, we need equal amounts. Some researchers suggest we may require twice as much Omega 6 as Omega 3. Unfortunately, the current Western diet results in deficiencies of both and what's more, the ratio is more likely to be 1:20 in favour of Omega 6.

Foods containing Omega 3 fats

- Flaxseeds (linseeds)
- Pumpkin seeds
- Hemp seeds
- Walnuts
- Oily fish such as salmon, sardines, mackerel
- Tuna
- Eggs

Foods containing Omega 6 fats

- Sunflower seeds
- Sesame seeds
- Pumpkin seeds
- Soya beans
- Maize
- Wheatgerm

Key points

- Reduce the amount of saturated fats in your diet
- Try to eliminate consumption of hydrogenated fats as far as possible
- Do make use of the nuts and seeds described in this chapter
- Use only extra virgin olive oil or coconut oil for frying and cooking
- Purchase supplements manufactured by reputable companies
- Use a little butter for spreading. In moderation it is actually healthier than most margarines because the latter often contain damaged fats
- The best margarines are those made with cold pressed oils that have not been processed. Vitequell is the brand recommended by most nutritional practitioners
- As a healthy alternative, use nut and seed butters as spreads. Pumpkin seed butter, for example, provides a reasonable balance between Omega 3 and Omega 6 fats. Explore what is available from your local health food store or supermarket
- Incorporate into your diet cold pressed unprocessed oils that are blended to provide a good balance between

Omega 3 and Omega 6 fatty acids. These oils can be used to make a salad dressing, or can be added to yoghurts and cooked dishes that are ready to be served.

TOP TIP!

If you wish to speed up your metabolism, try taking 2–3 tablespoons flaxseed oil (linseed oil) a day with meals. Make sure you choose a brand that states 'cold pressed' on the label. The oil should be sold in an airtight bottle or container so that it is not exposed to light. It should also be stored in a fridge to protect against spoilage, since the essential fats in the oil are damaged by exposure to heat, light and air. You can also sprinkle the oil over your food if you prefer.

14

Boost your immune system

Our bodies are constantly assailed by a multitude of enemies including bacteria, viruses, parasites, fungi and a wide range of pollutants. Fortunately we all possess a major defence against this myriad of threats: the immune system. With a complex range of specialised cells at its disposal, the immune system is capable of apprehending foreign invaders and destroying them. The main 'highways' into the body are the lungs and the digestive tract. Our lungs act as the interface between the body and the outside air while the lining of the intestines acts as the interface between the body and ingested food and liquids.

Also within its structure is the so-called 'gut-associated immune system'. This system resembles a border patrol at the boundary between two countries. It only allows completely digested food particles such as amino acids and simple sugars to pass through the gut wall into the bloodstream, where they are transported around the body to the tissues where they are needed. So far so good you might think, but when incompletely digested foods get past the 'border patrol' (gut wall), they can trigger off immune reactions including allergies and intolerances. If the gut wall is damaged due to yeast overgrowth or some other factor (see also page xx), these larger food particles get into the bloodstream more easily. Remember, this condition is referred to as 'leaky gut syndrome'. In essence, when the immune system works well, we usually experience a good level of health. However, like all complex systems, it can be prone to malfunction.

In Chapter 11, I conveyed to you how important it is to minimise toxins in the body and to supply the immune system with the raw materials it needs in order to function normally. The importance of this can be summed up when we compare the following simple equations:

Poor nutrition + toxins = weakened immune system = food intolerances + weight gain.

Compare this to:

Good nutrition + low level of toxins = strong immune system = fewer food intolerances + weight loss.

In this chapter, I'm going to inform you of the dietary methods that can be followed to further boost your immune system and reduce the level of toxins in your body, the first of these being juicing.

Juicing: The key to a healthy immune system
If you want to strengthen your immune system, increase your resistance to disease, help protect yourself from pollution, regulate your weight and lower your risk of food allergies and intolerances then the juice habit can be one of your greatest

THE BIG FAT MYSTERY

allies! No, I'm not talking about the juices you buy in cartons from your local supermarket although some of these can be good. I'm referring to freshly prepared vitamin, mineral and enzyme-rich juices made in your very own juicer. If you don't own a juicer, then believe me, it could be one of the best health investments that you could possibly make!

What do juicers do?

Well, the obvious answer is that juicers extract juice from fruits and vegetables. However, some people get a little confused about the process and some even think that juicing is similar to blending. The big difference is that a juice extractor separates the juice from the fibre in fruit and vegetables. In comparison, as the name suggests, a blender simply liquidises fruit and soft vegetables such as tomatoes. When you liquidise fruit and vegetables, what you get is a drink that also contains fibre. The big advantage of separating the fibre from the juice is all the vitamins, minerals and enzymes become quickly absorbed by the body and this wouldn't happen with fibre present. So, whenever you drink a freshly prepared juice, you are quite literally ingesting one of nature's finest health cocktails.

Types of juicer

Quite simply, there are two basic types of juicer to choose from: the centrifugal juicer and the masticating juicer and these are described in detail below.

The centrifugal juicer: These juicers chop fruit and vegetables into small pieces and throw them against a spinning bowl-shaped sieve. In this way, the juice is filtered through the sieve and comes out of one outlet and the fibre is then ejected through another outlet. They are quick and easy to use because they can deal with quite large pieces of fruit and vegetables. Some health experts say that centrifugal juicers do not produce the best-quality juice because they generate heat and when you subject the 'live' enzymes and other nutrients to heat, some of the nutritional value is destroyed. Well, this is true but do not be put off because the juice is still full of goodness, especially if it is consumed in minutes of being extracted.

Like everything else, when it comes to selecting a good-quality machine, it is always worth paying a little extra for quality. Some of the best centrifugal juicers on the market are extremely quiet and have lower speed motors to minimise the damage to the nutrient value of the juice. In fact, the best have a twin-speed motor – the slower speed is for green leafy vegetables, cucumber, celery, etc. and the higher speed designed for carrots, beetroot, pears and apples, etc.

The masticating juicer: This type of juicer crushes the fruit/vegetables and the juice is forced through a cone-shaped sieve. Meanwhile, fibre is ejected in a sausage-shape at one end of the machine. The advantage of this kind of machine is that very little heat is produced. Consequently, the resulting juice is a little higher in nutritional value, particularly enzymes, which are sensitive to heat. Some of these juicers can also deal with wheatgrass, which is very popular with juicing enthusiasts these days. Mind you, I cannot imagine that many people will become hooked on the stuff – it is definitely an acquired taste!

The big disadvantage of this type of juicer is it that it is much slower than the centrifugal type and you have to cut up the fruit and vegetables into much smaller pieces before feeding them into the machine.

TOP TIP

When selecting a juicer, choose a model that is easy to clean and has a good-quality motor. It should also be efficient at extracting juice from both fruit and vegetables, with a wide spout at the top to accommodate whole apples, etc.

Types of juice: Fruit

Apples are regarded as a sub-acid fruit (in contrast, for example, with oranges and lemons which are high in citric acid – hence the reason why they are referred to as citrus fruits). Apple juice also contains pectin that can absorb fats and toxins from the food we eat while in transit in the digestive system. Apple juice is extremely versatile and will blend with lots of other juices including quite a few vegetable juices. So, if you're making a juice out of vegetables such as celery, cucumber and carrot, it is often good to add an apple to the recipe because it will make the juice a lot more palatable. Apples possess very good detoxifying properties and this is partly due to their malic acid content, which means this juice often features prominently in cleansing programmes. Incidentally, malic acid is beneficial to the body, which is the reason why cider vinegar, with its malic acid content, is much better for you than other vinegars, especially spirit and malt vinegars, which can be irritating to the mucous membranes that line the digestive system.

Apples are rich in beta-carotene, which is converted by the body into vitamin A. They also contain vitamins B, C and E, folic acid, biotin and calcium, chlorine, magnesium, phosphorous, potassium, copper and zinc minerals.

Apricot: The pale-orange colour of this delicious fruit is due to their high beta-carotene content. Apricots make a lovely sweet and aromatic juice that can easily be mixed with apple and other juices such as mango.

Rich in beta-carotene, apricots contain most of the B complex vitamins, vitamin C and calcium, chlorine, magnesium, phosphorous and potassium.

Blackberry: Blackberries make good juice for mixing with other juices such as apple. They are nature's gift and if picked away from roadsides and pesticide-sprayed fields, they provide a free source of organic juice which is rich in nutrients.

Blackberries are rich in most of the B vitamins, beta-carotene, vitamins C and E. They're also a good source of calcium, magnesium, phosphorous, potassium, sodium and sulphur.

Blackcurrant: Ah, how I remember as a young boy, carefully plucking the sun-ripened blackcurrants from the bush at the bottom of our garden in Sunderland! I can still recall the succulent flavour of the jet-black berries. Indeed, blackcurrants make a flavourful and rich juice that can be used as a mixer with other juices such as apple and pear. It's a great detoxifier and provides a valuable boost to the immune system.

Blackcurrants are one of nature's richest sources of vitamin C; they are also rich in beta-carotene and vitamin E, which are wonderful antioxidants. As far as their mineral content is concerned, they're a good source of calcium, magnesium, phosphorous, potassium, sodium and sulphur in addition to small amounts of iron.

Cherry: Cherries vary in colour and sweetness depending on the variety. When using them to make juice, slice them in half to remove the stones. This is a bit time-consuming but the end result is well worth it. You can add cherry juice to other fruit such as apples, pears and grape. Cherries have a reputation for helping with inflammatory conditions such as arthritis and gout. One particular variety, Montmorency, is reputed to be the best for gout, increasing energy levels and helping to boost the immune system. A friend had been able to discard his medication for gout since drinking Montmorency juice.

Cherries are a good source of beta-carotene, vitamins C and E, biotin and a number of B vitamins. They also provide us with a good supply of calcium, magnesium, potassium, sodium and sulphur in addition to smaller amounts of copper, iron, manganese and zinc.

Cranberry: Most of us are familiar with the cranberry juice that can be bought in cartons from supermarkets. Unfortunately, these drinks are also high in sugar and in some cases, they contain artificial sweeteners to counteract the rather tart flavour of the cranberries. With the addition of sugar, much of the health-giving properties of the berries are lost. However, if you add a handful or two of natural berries to other fruits that you are juicing, then the tartness of the berries is offset due to the content of the natural fruit sugars derived from such fruits as apples and pears. So, not only is this is a great way of drinking cranberry juice, it also ensures that the cranberries do not lose their therapeutic properties. Cranberries are commonly used to help overcome the effects of cystitis, which women in particular are sometimes prone to.

Cranberries are rich in beta-carotene, folic acid, vitamin C and traces of some B vitamins. They are also a good source of calcium, magnesium, potassium and sulphur.

Grape: Broadly speaking, there are two types of juice, namely white and red. For many years grapes have been held in high regard by natural therapists because of their curative properties. In fact, the grape cure has been used in clinics to cure ailments as diverse as kidney stones and even purportedly some cancerous conditions.

When preparing grapes for juicing, first remove the stalks but do leave in the pips. Because grapes are one of the most chemically sprayed fruits, it is best to purchase organically grown fruit, if possible.

Grapes are rich in vitamins C and E and have traces of B1, B2 and B3. They are particularly high in potassium and this may account for their curative properties and good effects on kidney functioning. The juice is also a good source of calcium and magnesium.

Kiwi fruit: This makes a tangy-tasting juice that is good for mixing with other juices. Once you have peeled the fruit, simply feed into the machine along with such fruits as apples and pears. Kiwi fruit is known to be one of the fruits most likely to provoke an allergic response in some people. However, it is very nutritious, with one of the highest sources of vitamin C of any fruit.

As well as vitamin C, kiwi fruit is a good source of beta-carotene, along with smaller amounts of some B vitamins and calcium, magnesium, potassium, phosphorous and sodium, in addition to small amounts of iron.

Lemon: Lemon juice is very acidic, which gives it the sharp taste. It is very good as a mixer with sub-acid fruits such as apples and pears. Use only in small amounts, though –it can be a bit overpowering. Lemons are the only fruit permitted on an anti-Candida diet because their low sugar content doesn't feed yeast. Also excellent as a detoxifier!

Lemons are renowned for being a good source of vitamin C. What's more, the white pith surrounding the juicy flesh is high in bioflavenoids. These two nutrients work together and have powerful antioxidant properties. Lemon juice is also a good source of minerals, particularly calcium, magnesium and sulphur.

Melon (various types): Melons produce an aromatic and refreshing juice that is quickly absorbed by the body. This is the reason why melon juice is best drunk on its own because it is thought that its rapid absorption may impede the absorption of nutrients from other fruits if consumed at the same time.

Melons are rich in beta-carotene and other health-giving carotenes, which is why they are so richly coloured. They also contain lots of vitamin C, folic acid and the minerals calcium, chlorine, magnesium and potassium plus small amounts of iron and zinc. They also contain sulphur, which is said to be good for normal formation of healthy joints in developing children, in addition to being important in helping the body to detoxify itself.

Orange: Orange juice tends to be very popular with children but as with all acidic fruits, it is best to encourage your child to drink the juice through a straw to protect their teeth from erosion as a result of coming into contact with the fruit acids. Orange juice is good for us adults too, especially when mixed with other juices or equally delicious on its own. To prepare, just peel the oranges and cut into chunks for juicing.

Freshly made orange juice is far superior to shop-bought

varieties, especially the juices that have been made from concentrate. This means they have been diluted with mains water, which contains chemicals such as chlorine. Furthermore, all shop-bought juices are pasteurised, which means they are heated briefly to a high temperature to destroy any bacteria that may reduce the shelf-life of the juice. This process inevitably destroys nutrients, especially vitamin C. When you juice your own oranges you are getting nothing else but the pure juice with its vitamin C content more or less intact. As with lemons, when you juice the pith surrounding the flesh, you also derive bioflavonoids from the oranges too. Orange juice is also a good source of beta-carotene, some B vitamins, vitamin E and calcium, magnesium, phosphorous, potassium and smaller quantities of iron, manganese and zinc.

Pear: Pear juice is mild-tasting and a very versatile juice that mixes well with other juices, particularly apple. Due to its high pectin content, it is one of the best urinary and gastrointestinal cleansers. Drinking freshly-made pear juice diluted with a little pure water after a digestive upset can be soothing for your digestive system and it is also beneficial in terms of lowering your allergic potential.

Again, as with many fruits, pear is rich in beta-carotene, which is converted by the body into vitamin A. Vitamin A is needed to maintain the normal health of the mucous membranes lining the inner body surfaces – for example, the digestive tract and the lungs and wind-pipe (trachea). Pear juice also contains significant amounts of folic acid and vitamin C, as well as the minerals calcium, magnesium and potassium. The latter is very important for keeping the blood alkaline, which it needs to be in healthy adults and children.

Types of juice: Vegetables

Beetroot: This juice can only be taken in small quantities and certainly no more than a wine glassful to begin with. It should be mixed with other vegetable juices such as carrot, celery and apple to make it more palatable. Although beetroot is a powerful liver cleanser (and therefore favoured in natural cancer cures), it can actually make you feel quite nauseous if you drink too much of it. You can increase the quantity as you get used to it. Beetroot is excellent for building good healthy blood and for strengthening the immune system largely due to its high mineral content.

Beetroot is high in folic acid and vitamin C, as well as being rich in calcium, magnesium, potassium and phosphorous with lesser amounts of iron, zinc and copper.

Broccoli: This juice is quite strong and should always be mixed with other juices in small amounts. It is one of the richest sources of antioxidants and other nutrients, and is therefore one of the most powerful immune boosters.

Broccoli juice is rich in chlorophyll, which is believed to have therapeutic qualities. It is also a good source of protective antioxidants such as beta-carotene and vitamin C, as well as minerals, particularly calcium, magnesium, phosphorous and potassium.

Cabbage: Many people are surprised that cabbage juice has such a pleasantly sweet taste. It can easily be mixed with other juices like apple, celery and carrot. You can also add a small piece of ginger to give the juice an extra zing.

Cabbage juice has a reputation for healing stomach ulcers and it is thought to be good for the digestive system. Perhaps this may partly explain why cabbage and other members of the cruciferous family, such as cauliflower and broccoli, are believed to exert a protective effect against stomach and bowel cancer. Remember, also, that foods that have a healing effect on the lining of the digestive tract are likely to reduce your allergic potential.

Cabbage is high in vitamin C, folic acid and lesser amounts of some B vitamins, vitamin E and the minerals calcium, chlorine, magnesium, potassium and phosphorous.

Carrot: This is one of the richest sources of beta-carotene, which is converted into vitamin A by the body. Recent research suggests there may be a link between high-intake of this nutrient and the prevention of some types of cancer.

Many adults and children like the sweet taste of carrot juice but even those who don't enjoy it on its own can find it quite palatable when juiced with apple. Carrot juice forms the basis for many juicing detoxification programmes because it is very cleansing for the liver.

As well as being rich in beta-carotene, carrots are a good source of calcium, iron, magnesium and sodium.

Celery: This juice contains an abundance of organic sodium, an element good for the joints. Celery juice is also an excellent cleanser. It mixes very well with other vegetables such as cucumber, apple and carrot. Because it acts as a diuretic, it is also good for reducing water retention. Due to its low calorific content, celery juice is good when included in a weight-loss programme.

In addition to sodium, celery is rich in magnesium, calcium, iron and the vitamins folic acid and vitamin C. It also contains smaller amounts of some B vitamins and vitamin E.

Cucumber: Cucumber juice is refreshing in hot weather because it is very cooling. Combined with carrot and celery, it is said to be good for the hair and nails and for strengthening the immune system, perhaps because it is a good cleansing juice. Also, being low in calories, it is a brilliant juice to include in any weight-loss programme.

When I mention cucumbers to people they often remark, 'But they're mostly just water, aren't they?' True, they do have a high water content but they are surprisingly rich in calcium, chlorine, magnesium, potassium, sodium, sulphur and silicon. Cucumbers are also a good source of folic acid and vitamin C. Their high potassium content makes them a useful alkaline-forming juice.

Tomato: Tomato juice has a good cleansing action but only when consumed in the absence of concentrated starches such those present in bread and cereals.

Rich in vitamin C and beta-carotene, tomato juice is also a very good source of lycopene, a natural compound believed to exert a protective effect against some cancers. Tomatoes also provide a good supply of magnesium, potassium, sodium and calcium.

Juice recipes

As well as being an excellent source of nutrients, these juice recipes are a good addition to a weight loss programme, especially when used to provide you with energy between meals. In this regard, the recipes based mostly on vegetables are best because they often contain less sugar. Remember, when your energy levels are steady you're less likely to snack on the wrong types of food. Unless otherwise stated, all recipes serve one.

Lemon Sparkler

This juice is a great alternative to shop-bought lemonade – and much healthier too!

2 whole apples
I lemon
½ glass sparkling spring water

Juice the apple and lemon. Pour into a suitable container and top up with sparkling spring water.

Omega Fat Burner

This is a great juice for supplying those essential Omega 3 and Omega 6 fatty acids that are so crucial for a healthy immune system and for helping to burn up fat in the body. You might also remember from Chapter 13 on healthy fats that Omega 3 fatty acids are really good for increasing your metabolic rate. Higher Nature's Essential Balance oil and Udo's Choice oil are mixtures of Omega 3, 6 and 9 fats that are available from health food shops.

2 whole apples
2 carrots, peeled
I tsp of Higher Nature's Essential Balance oil or Udo's Choice oil

Juice the apples and carrots. Gently stir in the oil into the juice. Serve immediately.

Cucumber Cool

This juice is great for hot sunny days, mainly because of the addition of the cucumber, which is very cooling and cleansing.

½ cucumber
3 apples
2 sticks celery
2 carrots
ice, to serve
1 mint sprig, optional

Simply juice the fruit and vegetables together and serve in a tall glass with ice and a sprig of mint, if liked.

Lemon and Ginger Zinger
Ginger is a great pick-me-up and good for the digestion.

¼ pineapple, peeled and sliced
1 apple or pear
½ lemon
1 kiwi fruit
1cm (½in) piece of ginger

Juice all the ingredients, adding the ginger last of all. Stir the resulting juice and serve.

Red Alert!
The beetroot in this combo makes it a great for blood-building and detoxifying. it's also another valuable immune-booster.
1 beetroot
2 carrots
2 apples
1 stick celery

Peel the beetroot and carrots. Juice with the apples and celery, pour into a glass and serve.

Spicy Apple

1 lime
2 apples
1 tsp ground mixed spices

With a sharp knife, remove the peel from the lime to leave only the pith. Juice together with the apples and serve sprinkled with sweet spices.

Creamy Carrot

The addition of soya milk to carrot juice makes a lovely creamy drink that is a good source of protein with lots of beta-carotene, which is good for your immune system.

3 carrots
soya milk, to taste

Juice the carrots, stir in the soya milk and serve.

Fantastic Four!

This juice is packed full of vitamins and minerals. It is very cleansing for the liver and kidneys.

2 carrots
2 sticks of celery
1 small beetroot
2 tomatoes
ice cubes, to serve

Juice all of the vegetables together and serve with ice cubes –
very refreshing!

Popeye

The spinach in this recipe can only be juiced if you own a
juicer that can handle leafy vegetables. By alternating the
order in which the ingredients are added to the juicer,
making a kind of sandwich with the spinach as the filling, the
green spinach juice is extracted more efficiently.

2 apples
a handful of baby spinach
2 carrots
⅓ cucumber

With the juicer switched off, place an apple in the spout,
followed by half the spinach and half the cucumber. Switch
on and juice, then repeat with the remaining ingredients.

Banana Surprise

You'll just love the fruity flavours! This is also a great energy
booster and full of vitamin C.

1 peach
175g/6oz/1 cup strawberries, hulled
½ medium mango
1 pear
1 banana

Juice the peach, strawberries, mango and pear. Pour the juice into a blender then blend with the banana and serve.

Apple and Orange
This makes a very invigorating and refreshing drink. It is particularly good as a breakfast drink to give you extra energy in the mornings.

2 oranges
2 apples

Peel the oranges, leaving on the pith. Juice with the apples and serve.

Green Machine
Broccoli contains many valuable natural cancer-preventative compounds including indole-3-carbinol, which helps to protect us from harmful pollution.

2 apples
3 carrots
5 broccoli florets
5 lettuce leaves

Juice all the ingredients together and serve chilled.

Acidophilus Delight

This includes acidophilus powder (available from health food shops), which helps promote the balance of healthy bacteria in the gut.

1 apple
1 pear
1 kiwi fruit
8 grapes
1 carrot
½ tsp acidophilus powder

Juice the fruit and the carrot. Then stir in the acidophilus powder and serve.

Melon Medley

This delightful juice is full of vitamin C and beta-carotene, which are great for the immune system.

½ lemon
1 slice of watermelon, cut into chunks
1 pear
1 slice of honeydew melon, cut into chunks

Remove the rind from the lemon and feed into the juicer, then add the other ingredients.

Vegetable Cocktail

This juice is brimming with anti-oxidants, which help to protect the body from free-radicals (unstable molecules which have a destructive affect on the cells). They are produced as a result of metabolism and exposure to pollution.

2 tomatoes
2 sticks of celery
½ beetroot
I carrot
I bulb of fennel
2 apples

Juice all the ingredients together and drink immediately.

Smoothies

Most adults and children really love smoothies and although not as beneficial as freshly extracted juices, they are still a good source of nutrients.

Banana and Pineapple

¼ pineapple
I banana
3 tbsp bio-yoghurt or soya milk
Remove the skin from the pineapple and cut into chunks and juice. Place the other ingredients in a blender and blend until creamy and smooth. Stir in the pineapple and serve.

Banana, Peach and Strawberries

Children and adults alike love the combined flavours of this creamy smoothie.

1 peach
1 banana
10 strawberries, hulled
3 tbsp bio-yoghurt or soya milk

Remove the stone from the peach and cut into chunks. Cut the banana into slices. Place all the fruit in a blender and stir in the yoghurt or soya milk last of all. Serve.

Coconut Delight

1 mango
1 kiwi fruit
3 apricots
225ml/8 floz/1 cup canned coconut milk

Peel the mango, remove the stone and cut into pieces. Then peel the kiwi fruit and cut into slices. Blend with the apricots, adding the coconut milk until creamy and smooth.

Berry Delight

A very popular, brightly coloured smoothie that tastes as delicious as it looks, too! Blueberries can be purchased frozen, or you can freeze fresh ones by placing them on a tray for an hour in the freezer, then transferring them to a suitable container, where they will keep for about a month.

1 apple
a handful of frozen blueberries
1 frozen banana
a handful of frozen strawberries
1 kiwi fruit
225ml/8 fl oz/1 cup soya milk

Place all the ingredients in a blender and blend until a thick, creamy consistency is achieved. Serve.

Brain Booster

This is a good way of providing essential fatty acids for normal brain functioning and a healthy immune system.

1 apple
165g/5½oz/1 cup melon pieces
1 peach
225g/8oz/1 cup ready frozen raspberries
2 apricots
1 tbsp Higher Nature's Essential Balance or Udo's Choice oil (from
    health shops)
3 ice cubes

Blend the fruit and ice cubes until creamy smooth and drizzle in the oil; blend for a few seconds and serve.

15

The power of living foods

Let me begin this chapter with a question: what do vegetables, grains, and nuts sprouted from seeds have in common? Answer: they are all living foods. Living foods are high in vitamins, minerals, phytonutrients and enzymes. These are components of uncooked foods that are crucial to the maintenance of good health. It has been a central theme of this book that each and every one of the billions of cells that make up the human body needs these vital components to function at optimal level. In essence, if your cells are functioning well, then *you* function well! Conversely, it only takes the cellular make-up of one organ system in the body to malfunction – for example, the liver – and the end result is the manifestation of illness. As I've already stated, most experts within the field of natural health agree that normal cellular function is comprised of a build-up of toxicity within the body in addition to nutritional imbalances and deficiencies. The best way to supply the body with these vital nutrients in their correct balance is to live on the natural and vibrant foods that nature has provided for us. This helps to ensure that the body does not become over-burdened by an excess of toxins.

Over the years many natural health pioneers have discovered the powerful healing effects of living foods. Some of them, such as Dr Bircher-Benner, set up clinics in order to treat the chronically sick, often with great success. He was head of the Life-Force Sanitorium (on the slopes of the Zurichberg outside Zurich, Switzerland) in the late nineteenth century, and is known for his ground-breaking work with raw food nutritional therapy. He repeatedly observed in the course of his practice that a diet of wholesome uncooked food improved the health of many of his patients, some of whom were on the verge of death. In the early 1900s Dr Max Gerson first cured his own chronic migraines before using the same dietary principles to treat various diseases, from supposedly incurable conditions such as lupus to diabetes. He even cured Albert Schweitzer's wife of tuberculosis. Later he learned that living foods improve cellular function and respiration, as well as strengthening the immune system, thus encouraging the body to heal itself. Gerson discovered that a diet of natural, living foods in conjunction with copious amounts of freshly extracted organic fruit and vegetable juices could be used to successfully treat cancer and I believe that many people who have been stricken with cancer are alive today, possibly as a result of trying this therapy.

What are sprouts?

A good example of sprouts is the ones we all learned to grow from mustard and cress seeds when we were children. I'm sure that you too took great delight in watching the seeds gradually transform into green chlorophyll-filled shoots that soon developed into dozens of tiny little plants. This would usually take only a few days and the end result was delicious, fresh-tasting greens packed with nutrients. In much the same way, you can grow sprouts from alfalfa, broccoli, radish, fenugreek, red clover and onion seeds. In addition, pulses can be sprouted from mung beans, chickpeas and aduki beans. It is also possible to sprout grains such as wheat and barley. Both these grains mature into wheatgrass and barley grass respectively, which can be juiced and have powerful cleansing and healing properties. The good news for those people who are intolerant to the grains themselves is that the sprouts do not usually cause any problems. It is even possible to sprout nuts and seeds. One of the most popular nuts for sprouting is almonds and these are highly nutritious and easy to digest.

The thing that I find wonderful about seeds is that the 'life' in them lies dormant until sprouted when suddenly a living plant explodes into being. That is wonderful in itself, but just as amazing is that when seeds are sprouted, enzyme levels increase dramatically, proteins are converted to amino acids and simple carbohydrates (sugars) and vitamin and mineral levels are multiplied many times over. This means that sprouts are highly anti-oxidant and because of their high enzyme content, they are much easier to digest than most foods. So, for example, if someone has a problem with digesting pulses such as beans they may find that when these beans are sprouted, they can digest them without any problems. Sprouts are very versatile and can liven up sandwich fillings or be added to salad or juices.

How to sprout

Seeds have to be soaked before they will sprout. The basic rule is to base soaking times on the size of the seeds. As you might imagine, larger seeds need to be soaked for longer than small seeds:

- Small seeds: soak for 4–6 hours

- Medium seeds: soak for 8–10 hours
- Large seeds: soak for 12–24 hours

Nuts, seeds, grains and pulses must be placed in a glass or stainless steel container (avoid aluminium and plastic since they may contaminate the sprouts). They should then be covered with filtered water (two or three times as much water as seeds). This allows the contents enough room to expand. The following table shows the amount of seeds you need to use for sprouting, as well as soaking and sprouting time:

Type of seed	Soaking time	sprouting time	measure
HULLED SEEDS			
Pumpkin	4 hours	24 hours	1 cup
Seasame	4 hours	12 hours	1 cup
Sunflower	6 hours	24 hours	1 cup
GRANS (ALKALINE-FORMING)			
Amaranth	3 hours	24 hours	1 cup
Millet	6 hours	12 hours	1 cup
Quinoa	3 hours	24 hours	1 cup
LARGE GRAINS (ACID-FORMING)			
Barley	6 hours	12 hours	1 cup
Corn	12 hours	36 hours	1 cup
Spelt wheat	6 hours	36 hours	1 cup
Wheat	6 hours	36 hours	1 cup
VEGETABLES			
Alfalfa	5 hours	5 days	3tbsp
Broccoli	5 hours	5 days	3tbsp
Cabbage	5 hours	4–5 days	3 tbsp
Fenugreek	6 hours	5 days	¼cup
Kale	5 hours	5 days	¼cup
Mustard	5–6 hours	5 days	3tbsp
Radish	5–6 hours	5 days	3 tbps

PULSES

Aduki beans	5–6 hours	5 days	3tbsp
Chickpeas	12 hours	3 days	1 cup
Lentils – all types	8 hours	3 days	¾cup
Mung beans	8 hours	5 days	1 cup
Peas	8 hours	3 days	1½cups

Sprouting equipment

The most basic equipment comprises a glass jar and all you have to do to germinate your seeds, grains, pulses or nuts is to cover the requisite amount in pure water and soak for the necessary time (see table above). Afterwards, just pour off the cloudy water and rinse the seeds well. You will then need to fix some muslin or mesh over the mouth of the jar and place it upside down in a dish rack at a 45° angle in indirect sunlight to drain the water off. Then place the jar in a place where the seeds, etc. will be exposed to sunlight and rinse one or two times daily. When the seeds, nuts, etc. are fully sprouted, consume or dry; store them in the fridge until needed.

You can now buy a jar specifically designed for this purpose from a number of companies and one of the best is available from a company called Bioforce (see Useful Information, page 303). They also supply a sprouter consisting of several trays with drainage holes – good when you want to sprout several different sprouts at once. If you really get serious about sprouting, I suggest you buy an automatic sprouter that can accommodate several seed trays. A timer ensures that the seeds are automatically sprayed with water twice daily. You can even buy extra sections to hold more seed trays. Having said this, even if you decide to grow sprouts with just the basic equipment, this is still a marvellous way of growing your own nutrient-rich sprouts all year round. Just imagine being able to include sprouted nuts, seeds, grains and pulses in all your salads and sandwiches, knowing that you are feeding yourself with what amounts to the highest quality 'live' foods that are free from pesticides, fungicides and other potentially harmful chemicals.

A family-by-family guide to sprouting seeds

- *Leafy sprouts:* Alfalfa, cress, radish, fenugreek, clover
- *Sprouting pulses:* Mung, peas, lentils, chickpeas, aduki
- *Brassica sprouts:* Broccoli, radish, mustard, cress
- *Grains:* Wheat, spelt, quinoa, buckwheat, kamut (this ancient grain is a relative of modern wheat), rye
- *Sprout greens:* Sunflower, buckwheat lettuce, pea shoots
- *Nuts and seeds:* Almonds, pumpkin, hulled sunflower seeds, sesame
- *Alliums:* Garlic, onion, leek.

FOOD FACT

Anne Wigmore was a true pioneer of sprouting. She first discovered the amazing healing properties of sprouts after acquiring a pet monkey that had no teeth. She tried feeding it with seeds but these were too hard and so she placed them between wet towels to soften them. I think you can guess what happened next! Yes, the seeds began to sprout and after feeding them to the monkey, it quickly regained its health. What's more, Anne Wigmore herself was suffering from cancer and had tried unsuccessfully to cure herself using wheatgrass and unsprouted seeds, but then she hit upon something quite remarkable... When she began eating the sprouted versions of seeds such as sunflower, buckwheat and mung beans, she too began to get well.

16

Minimising your body's toxic load

When we are well nourished and living on a healthy diet, we are far less likely to suffer from the food cravings that can ultimately lead to weight gain. However, because we know that many toxins are anti-nutrients, we are also aware that they destroy the body's supply of vitamins and minerals. This is precisely why we must minimise exposure to the pollutants that we experience every day of our lives.

Keeping the body as free from internal pollution as possible is one of the cornerstones of an approach designed to increase our resistance to food allergies and intolerances and to free the obstacles that stand in the way of effective weight management. If we subscribe to the view that a clean internal environment, coupled with well-nourished cells, helps reduce our allergic potential, then we must think in terms of not only reducing the toxins produced as a result of a poor diet but also attempt to reduce those that enter our bodies in the form of external pollutants. To achieve this, it is imperative that we increase our awareness of the everyday sources of pollution to which we are exposed, only then can we make informed decisions about how to protect ourselves. Remember, permanent weight loss is the result of eradicating food allergens and balancing the whole body.

Sadly, every facet of our modern-day existence seems to be affected by one type of pollution or another. The fact that words such as 'global warming', 'carbon emissions', 'radioactive fall-out', 'pesticides', 'radiation', 'genetically modified crops', 'ozone and gender-bending chemicals' have become an integral part of our everyday vocabulary is very telling about the world in which we now live. Thankfully, an increasing number of people from around the world are becoming educated about the need to initiate changes, locally and globally. Meaningful worldwide debate is taking place to bring about positive change. Meanwhile, until such changes occur, what should we do? Should we just accept that it's OK to live in an environment forcing us to attempt to cope with the daily onslaught of chemical pollutants? Is it acceptable to then compound the problem by feeding ourselves (and our children) a less than adequate diet? Well, the bad news is that it's impossible to completely protect ourselves from the effects of environmental pollution. The good news, however, is that there is no reason for us to be helpless victims of a polluted environment because positive action can be taken that will afford us protection, especially with regard to healthy eating and sensible use of vitamin and mineral supplements.

Protection from pollution

The pre-requisite to protecting ourselves from the effects of pollution is to increase our awareness of the sources of pollutants in our environment. This being the case, the following information should prove invaluable.

Air pollution

Vehicle emissions are responsible for a significant amount of air pollution in developed countries. Exposure is usually higher in towns and cities. Also, if you live close to a main road with a high volume of traffic then pollution exposure will increase.

Exhaust fumes contain a variety of chemicals including benzene, nitrous oxide (a known lung irritant), carbon monoxide (odourless and colourless, poisonous gas), hydrocarbons and, to a lesser extent these days: lead. Diesel fumes emitted from diesel cars, lorries and buses tend to be higher in hydrocarbons, which are basically like air-born particles of soot. The effects of such air pollution have been linked to lung diseases, including bronchitis, lung cancer and asthma. Many scientists also believe thousands of fatalities each year can be attributed to air pollution from vehicle exhausts.

To minimise exposure, try to avoid walking along routes that involve being in close proximity to main roads. It is also a good idea to close car windows in heavy traffic (for example, when travelling through a tunnel). Some cars have an air re-circulation device that can be used for short periods while in heavy traffic. It is also possible to purchase air filters to improve the air quality in your home.

Tobacco smoke

This contains thousands of chemicals including the addictive compound nicotine, in addition to tar and cadmium. A lot of people mistakenly believe that the brown stains sometimes visible on the fingers of heavy smokers are nicotine. In fact, it is the tar in the cigarette smoke that stains the fingers brown. Nicotene is actually a clear oily substance that resembles colourless baby oil. It is thought to be one of the principle addictive chemicals found in tobacco smoke. Cadmium is a substance that has similar effects to lead. Both lead and cadmium can damage the nervous system and add to your body's toxic load.

Thankfully, exposure to other people's tobacco smoke is much less of a problem these days with the introduction of more and more no-smoking areas! This isn't good news for the smokers, but it's certainly better for our lungs. When I was a child I was exposed to an almost incessant cloud of cigarette smoke because both my parents were heavy smokers. Fortunately, most people are aware of the dangers associated with passive smoking and I would like to think that parents who smoke are now sensible enough to smoke away from the presence of their children.

Aerosols

I have always been a bit suspicious about breathing in the fumes from aerosols. Whether it's hairsprays, deodorants, fly sprays or insecticides, all contaminate our air with air-borne chemicals. These chemicals are breathed into our lungs, where they come into contact with mucous membranes that can be irritated by foreign chemicals. Such chemicals can also be absorbed into the body via the lungs and may trigger off allergies.

Try to avoid using aerosols in a confined space, such as your bathroom or living room. This is especially important if you are using any kind of pesticide such as fly-killer. When applying hair spray, make sure you keep the room well ventilated.

Heavy metals

When I was at school I was fascinated to discover that our world and everything in it is made from elements. Some of these, including calcium, carbon and oxygen, are essential for life. Nevertheless, I was equally fascinated to learn that some of these elements (such as lead, arsenic, cadmium and mercury) can be highly toxic to the body. Unfortunately, certain toxic elements are present in our everyday environment.

Lead:

With the advent of unleaded petrol, most lead pollution today comes from lead pipes in older houses. It is also sometimes found in paint, but not usually in modern paints. Lead has an adverse affect on the nervous system, particularly on the developing nervous systems of young children.

If you have lead pipes in your house it is important to turn on the tap first thing in the morning and allow the water to run for a couple of minutes to reduce the lead content. This is because lead will accumulate in the water system when in contact with the pipes overnight. Ideally, lead pipes should be replaced. Some people invest in a water filtration system to be installed in their house (see also page 266, later on in this chapter).

Cadmium:

As I've already stated above in the section on tobacco smoke, cadmium has similar effects to lead in that it can adversely affect brain development and lead to behavioural problems. Some environmentalists speculate that a combination of lead and cadmium could produce an even more potent affect on the central nervous system. Smokers are particularly susceptible to cadmium exposure because it is found in cigarettes. To minimise your exposure, try to limit your exposure to passive smoke.

Mercury

This is a highly toxic metal known to cause brain damage.

The expression 'Mad as a hatter' originates from the nineteenth century when hat-makers used mercury compounds to blacken top hats. In addition, mercury harms the digestive tract, nervous system and the kidneys and can result in birth defects.

Mercury gets into the human body through more than one source. One source is through the food chain. Being a by-product of certain industrial processes, mercury ends up in rivers from where it can eventually make its way into seas and oceans. It can therefore accumulate in fish, especially tuna, swordfish, mackerel and shark. For this reason, it may be advisable to limit your consumption to perhaps two or three times per week. Pregnant women in particular should be careful about their weekly intake because the developing foetus is extremely vulnerable to the effects of this heavy metal.

Over recent years there has been much controversy concerning mercury amalgam fillings. Dentists in the UK tend to adopt the stance that mercury poses no threat and state that once set, the amalgam is very stable. This view is challenged by some dentists and many natural therapists who deal in heavy metal contamination, however. Studies reveal that mercury amalgam, far from being the inert substance we were led to believe, is constantly eroded in the mouth. This happens, for example, when we drink something hot such as tea or coffee or when we eat certain foods that result in the conversion of the mercury into methyl mercury. Methyl mercury may be swallowed and absorbed through the gut; it can also be breathed in and enters the body via the lungs from whence it goes into the bloodstream.

Once mercury finds its way into the body, one way that the body deals with it is to store it in fat cells. So, fatty tissues are a prime dumping ground for mercury. This is one of the reasons why mercury can exert toxic effects on the central nervous system because the brain is largely made up of fats. Certainly, convincing anecdotal evidence exists to show that when mercury is removed from the body, chronic conditions such as ME have been known to disappear. Crazy as it sounds, mercury has been used as one of the components in vaccine serum. Fortunately, it would appear that this is now becoming less common.

Aside from limiting your intake of tuna fish, I suggest any new dental fillings that you may need should be the white variety. These fillings do not last as long as mercury, nor are they completely non-toxic since they are made from a plastic composite which can include fillers to add strength and durability. Nevertheless, I suggest they are a much safer alternative to mercury amalgam. I feel that it's also advisable to replace worn-out or broken mercury fillings with white fillings whenever possible and usually dentists will give you the choice. Some people decide to have all of their amalgam removed and replaced with safer fillings. I must stress this should be carried out by a reputable dentist who uses specialised techniques to prevent the mercury released from the amalgam being absorbed into the body. Usually, post-dental treatment involves mineral chelation therapy. What happens is that the chelated minerals, such as zinc, bind onto the mercury until it is excreted from the body and this procedure needs to be carried out by a practitioner experienced in using this approach.

Aluminium:

This is a metal that can be absorbed into the body via food, water, air or skin contact. A common source of aluminium toxicity is aluminium cookware such as pots and pans. This kind of cookware is particularly dangerous because aluminium is a soft metal that is also water-soluble, which means the metal is released into the cooking water and easily mixes with your food.

To compound the problem, a number of water companies add aluminium to the water supply as a cleanser. It is also present in a wide range of products including deodorants, toothpaste, baking powder, aluminium foil, table salt (check the ingredients), dried milk, tea bags and some antacid remedies.

Research into loss of memory and Alzheimer's disease began in the 1960s. Although the connection between aluminium and Alzheimer's disease is yet to be proven, aluminium patches of cell damage in the brain known as plaques have been discovered in the brains of sufferers. This would certainly appear to suggest that aluminium may be implicated in the disease.

To minimise your exposure to this metal I would recommend you implement the following:

- Avoid using aluminium cookware – use stainless steel instead
- Avoid using the raising agent sodium aluminium phosphate (listed as additive E541). Scrutinise food labels on packets of biscuits and cakes that may contain this additive
- Avoid using antacids which contain aluminium hydroxide. Explore the use of natural alternatives instead.
- Avoid cooking (and wrapping) foods in aluminium foil
- Where possible avoid tap water. Use filtered or spring water instead
- Choose aluminium-free deodorants.

Heavy metal protection plan
Ensure that your diet includes the following:

- *Heavy metal antagonists:* These include vitamin C and calcium, magnesium, selenium and zinc. These nutrients are also available from green leafy vegetables, fresh fruit, nuts and seeds
- *Foods rich in pectin:* This binds the toxic metals and allows them to be excreted. Pectin is found in fresh fruits such as apples, bananas, pears and plums
- Foods such as pulses, seeds, white meat, fish and wholegrains
- Supplement your diet with a broad spectrum vitamin and mineral supplement (for recommended companies, see Useful Information, page 303).

Water
Sadly, as with many other natural resources today, water isn't what it used to be. The drinking water from your tap now contains a number of pollutants and these may exceed current safety levels. Some of these chemicals – for instance, nitrates and heavy metals such as lead – may represent a threat to your health. Other chemicals such as fluoride and chlorine are purposefully added to the water supply.

The pros and cons of fluoride
Fluoride is added to water as a means of reducing tooth decay. At levels of one part per million (1PPM), the evidence suggests that fluoride does indeed reduce tooth decay. However, conversely, at a level of 2PPM it can cause a mottling of the teeth known as fluorosis. In addition to this form of mass medication, we also ingest fluoride from other sources such as toothpaste and dental treatments.

Although the amount of fluoride added to water supplies is small, the amount absorbed by individuals can be variable. For example, it is known that you will absorb more fluoride if you reside in a soft water area because soft water provides an acid medium. No doubt the debate about the safety of fluoride as a water additive will continue for some time. However, I am a great believer in erring on the side of caution when it comes to ingesting substances that could be potentially be harmful to health, hence the reason for minimising exposure to fluoride as much as possible.

MINIMISE YOUR INTAKE OF FLUORIDE
Avoid drinking tap-water as much as possible
Use pure filtered water or spring water whenever possible

Chlorine

The addition of chlorine to water supplies is widely accepted. Unfortunately, it is known that chlorine can react with other substances such as peat that are also present in water. This results in the formation of chloroform, which has been linked with the formation of some cancers, including colon cancer. I would strongly advise you to avoid Jacuzzis, where chemicals such as chlorine are used to kill bacteria. The combination of aerating bubbles and hot water releases more chlorine into the air, which you then breathe in.

Minimise your intake of chlorine by following the same guidance for avoiding fluoride.

Nitrates

Farmers used to rely on good old-fashioned manure to fertilise their crops. Today there's a great dependency upon nitrogen based fertilisers. However, if such fertilisers are used in excessive quantities then the crops cannot absorb the entire amount of nitrate that is produced. The end result is that surplus nitrates are washed into streams, rivers and underground reservoirs, all of which can be a source of drinking water.

Excessive nitrates in water can damage the environment. They are also linked to ill health in humans because they are known to form nitrosamines, which are recognised as being potentially carcinogenic. Other potentially harmful substances that often find their way into our water supply include:

- Pesticides
- Silage and slurry
- Dioxins – a by-product from bleaching paper products and other manufacturing processes
- Phosphates from detergent washing powders
- Lead, particularly when old lead pipes are used to channel domestic water.

Of course, all of this makes grim reading. However, if you are serious about protecting yourself from pollution, the following options are worth considering.

Bottled water

Consumption of bottled water in the UK has rapidly increased over recent years. Most bottled waters come from pure underground sources, having first been filtered through several types of rock strata, sometimes over many years.

Filtered water

Some people opt for plumbed-in water filters. Once installed, a separate tap provides filtered water. Filters consist of carbon that filters out water impurities such as chlorine and lead. It's advisable to change filters regularly because they can turn into a breeding ground for bacteria.

The other option is the plastic jug type of filter, which again uses activated carbon. These filters need to be changed regularly according to the manufacturer's instructions.

Distilled water

This is very pure, soft water but in terms of taste, it tends to be inferior to natural spring water. Also, spring water can be a good source of trace minerals while water that has been distilled has had its minerals removed. Although not as good as bottled water, I feel that distilled water is still superior to tap water and provided that a natural diet is adhered to, an adequate supply of minerals should be available to the body.

Reverse osmosis filters

This type of filter removes a lot of impurities, including bacteria, viruses, aluminium, heavy metals and fluoride. However, the process involved can be rather wasteful in terms of the quantity of water required to produce acceptable drinking water. Distillers also use lots of electricity.

For those of you who decide to use mains water, it is worth taking the following precautions:

- When you turn on a tap for drinking water, allow the water to run for a couple of minutes to help dissipate impurities that have built-up in lead or copper pipes overnight.

- Don't use hot water directly from the tap for consumption – it is more likely to dissolve aluminium from your immersion heater, and copper and lead from pipes.
- Ensure you take a broad spectrum vitamin and mineral supplement (see Useful Information, page 303). Minerals such as calcium and magnesium exert a protective effect against aluminium and fluoride.
- Supplementing your diet with vitamin C offers protection against the formation of nitrosamines (see Nitrates, above).

How to avoid common food products and artificial additives that may add to your toxic load

When you think about it, the consumption of artificial additives may add to the toxins that our bodies have to deal with. Let's face it: it's easy to be misled about the ingredients listed on some food products. Many of them are best avoided in the interests of reducing our intake of toxins because often they are refined and therefore classed as anti-nutrients. For instance, as already stated, white sugar and white flour are classed as anti-nutrients because they use up the body's supply of vitamins and minerals in the digestive process. The following list of labels will help you discern the good from the bad when scrutinising products.

Wheat flour: This is just another name for white flour. Using the word 'wheat' instead of 'white flour' fools some shoppers into thinking it is whole wheat.

Organic wheat flour: Again, this is simply white flour. Just because it is derived from wheat that has been grown organically does not mean it is healthy.

Sucrose: This is just the scientific name for white or brown sugar, which as stated earlier in this book, should be avoided whenever possible.

White sugar: Speaks for itself!

Cane sugar: Just another name for white sugar. Remember, if it says 'organic cane sugar', it's still 'refined sugar'.

Sugar syrup: Guess what? Yes, that's right: this is just a liquid version of the white stuff!

Brown sugar: Just because it's brown doesn't mean that it's healthy! Brown sugar comes in different shades according to how refined it is. The crudest types such as dark muscovado and molasses do contain some minerals and so they are better for us than the more refined types. This is why I have included small amounts of the less refined sugars in the recipes in Part I of this book.

High fructose corn syrup, maltose, glucose, dextrose, lactose and fructose: All simple sugars and therefore elevate blood sugar levels. This is bad news for people who wish to lose weight because fluctuating blood sugar levels result in cravings for more refined carbohydrates that feed your need for another quick energy fix. High fructose corn syrup is now used as an ingredient in lots of products because it is a cheap option for manufacturers.

Granary bread: A lot of people are fooled by this one: granary bread is just white bread coloured brown with malt! It quickly elevates blood sugar levels and uses up the body's nutrients just like any other refined carbohydrate. For this reason, along with white bread, it's definitely on the forbidden list when it comes to any weight-loss programme. The only exception to the rule is if you can find a version using 100% wholewheat flour as the main ingredient.

Monosodium glutamate (MSG): This is an additive added to a multitude of foods today. It is a well-known ingredient in Chinese meals and is used to enhance flavour. MSG is commonly found in many savoury snacks that are popular with children. It is implicated in a number of health conditions including a possible cause of migraines in some and so my advice is to avoid feeding yourself and your children with food products that contain it whenever possible. It is possible to purchase savoury snacks that are naturally flavoured from your local health food shop or the healthy section of your supermarket.

Aspartame: This artificial sweetener is implicated in a number of health conditions including Pre-Menstrual Syndrome (PMS) and depression.

Hydrogenated oil (or partially hydrogenated oil): This is known as a trans fat, which is unnatural to the body (see Chapter 13, page 221). It also competes with good fats in the body and is linked with heart disease.

Cooking oils such as sunflower and safflower: The fact is that these should never be used for cooking because when subjected to heat (for example, when frying), the polyunsaturated fats they contain become damaged and they then become destructive fats. Moreover, manufacturers do not tell you that these oils are often extracted using chemical processes. They are also usually subjected to heat and light that further damages the healthy fats (see also, *Fats That Heal, Fats That Kill* by Udo Erasmus, page 302).

Artificial colours: These are used to artificially colour foods to make them look more attractive. They can be found in a wide range of foods so be on your guard! I'm sure you wouldn't dream of putting artificial dyes into your food at home when preparing meals, so my advice is to avoid these like the plague.

Artificial flavours: These are chemical additives that are designed to get you hooked. Like artificial colours, they are often linked with health problems, including mood swings and hyperactivity in children.

Genetically modified (GM) foods: GM foods are made from plants that have had their DNA changed to create certain characteristics such as longer shelf-life or more disease-resistant crops. However, most people are unhappy about their possible long-term effects on health and choose to avoid them. Unless you are happy for you and your children to become human guinea pigs, I would advise you to do the same!

Artificial preservatives: As the name suggests, these are designed to preserve food, thus extending shelf-life. They work because they kill the micro-organisms that thrive on food – for example, moulds and certain bacteria. Logic dictates that if they will destroy these forms of life, then they can't be good for the cells in our bodies. Watch out for sodium benzoate (E211), a commonly used preservative in carbonated drinks, too.

Sodium nitrite: This is an additive in foods such as bacon, ham and frankfurter sausages. It is used to impart an attractive red colour. My advice is to avoid it. Studies have indicated that it forms chemicals known as nitrosamines in the stomach and these are known to be carcinogenic. When I inform people about nitrites they are shocked because they frequently use ham in their sandwiches or in salads.

Raising agents: Used for baking, avoid those containing aluminium because it has been associated with Alzheimer's disease (see also page 261). For the same reason, you are advised to avoid using cooking utensils made of aluminium.

Glazing agents: These are used to impart a shiny coating, such as wax on oranges and lemons, so whenever possible, select non-waxed fruit.

Cosmetic ingredients

Take a look at the list of ingredients used to make many cosmetic products and more often than not you will see a wide range of chemical additives, many of them with unpronounceable names. Some of these ingredients have already been banned in certain countries because their safety is in question. They are thought to cause skin irritation, allergic reactions and may even be carcinogenic. At one time, despite being careful to avoid additives in my diet, I was totally ignorant of the fact that I was using products such as shampoos and skin creams that are packed with chemical additives. This changed one day when someone who had studied the subject asked me, 'Dave, you don't eat junk foods, so why would you want to absorb junk through your skin?' Point taken! I have since discovered that chemicals are indeed absorbed through the medium of the skin because this organ is a semi-permeable layer. This is aptly illustrated when you consider that if you rub a clove of garlic on the soles of your feet, later you will also smell garlic on your breath.

Some people do become sensitive to chemicals in cosmetics and household cleaning products. I once came across a client who, having been tested for environmental sensitivities, showed a positive reaction to the chemicals used in the manufacture of cotton T-shirts. When he changed to another material his skin condition cleared up. Now, I'm not saying you have to be obsessed about avoiding every product on the market – I'm sure some products, such as children's shampoos, will be purer than others. However, I think it pays to be discerning so I advise you to look out for the worst additives and try to purchase products that use safer alternatives. For a list of reputable manufacturers who use pure natural ingredients, please refer to Useful Information, page 301 at the back of this book.

The foregoing list of additives represents a general guide only. Should you wish to delve into the subject further, however, I recommend that you purchase a book on the subject to use as a quick reference guide should you be unsure about a particular ingredient – for example, artificial colours and flavours. A book that I particularly recommend is *The Chemical Maze Shopping Companion* (see page 302). This is a very comprehensive pocket-sized guide to the vast array of additives used in foods and also those included in cosmetics.

17

Healing the gut: the last piece of the weight-loss jigsaw

So far in this book I've addressed some key factors which, singly or combined, can exert a significant impact on your attempts to lose those excess pounds. You'll now be aware that the digestive system is pretty much a major area when it comes to influencing weight. When the gut lining is inflamed there is a greater chance that you will develop a leaky gut along with a greater sensitivity towards everyday foods. Therefore, in addition to devoting your attention to following a healthy diet and so minimising your intake of toxins, healing the gut and reducing inflammation represents the final piece of the weight loss jigsaw. In so doing, we may achieve the following:

- Our propensity to develop food intolerances is reduced
- Symptoms of intolerances are alleviated
- Our chances of reversing any food sensitivities are reversed
- Welcome relief to an over-stressed immune system is provided
- Our ability to regulate body weight is increased.

Alleviating the symptoms of food intolerance

As discussed in Chapter 3, IgG antibodies combine with offending foods (allergens) and may result in delayed immune responses in the body. Conversely, IgE reactions result in an immediate immune response – for example, someone who is allergic to apples may experience swollen lips and a sore throat as soon as an apple is eaten. The ensuing symptoms are the result of the release of histamine in the body. The same thing can happen in the digestive tract causing immediate gastric distress. It's the histamine that causes inflammation and swelling of the body's tissues. Whether the release of histamine is immediate or delayed, it is known that certain natural substances are capable either of dampening down the histamine releasing mechanism or they may help to reduce the inflammation resulting from histamine release. Some of these substances have a dual function in that they reduce inflammation and also help to heal the lining of the digestive tract. Below is a list of some of the most recommended supplements.

Omega 3 essential fats

As discussed in Chapter 13, Omega 3 fats are converted into hormone-like substances known as prostaglandins by the body. They are processed into series three prostaglandins, which have an anti-inflammatory effect in the body. The best sources are fish oils or oils extracted from flaxseed (linseed).

Methyl-Sulfonyl-Methane (MSM)

MSM is a natural substance found in plants and animals. It is a rich supply of sulphur, a mineral which is part of the structure of over 150 compounds including sulphurous amino acids, proteins, collagen, skin, nails, antibodies, enzymes and hormones. It's also a vital component of the body's most powerful antioxidant, the enzyme glutathione.

Antioxidants help protect us from unstable molecules known as free-radicals which can damage cells.

It appears that if we eat natural foods the level of MSM that we ingest on a daily basis is around 1mg MSM per kilo of body weight. Hence, if you are a man weighing 80kg (176lb), this amounts to 80mg, of which about one third is elemental (pure) sulphur. However, some MSM is lost as a result of excessive cooking and by eating too many processed foods hence the reason for supplementation.

In terms of allergies and food intolerances, MSM appears to have a significant anti-inflammatory action, largely because of the following:

- It coats the lining of the small intestine which may help to alleviate inflammation
- MSM may help to reverse a leaky gut because it exerts a healing effect on the gut lining. This in turn has the potential to alleviate food related immune responses in the body
- It provides intestinal bacteria with the components they need to manufacture allergy-fighting amino acids such as cysteine and methionine
- In terms of its ability to reduce allergic responses to food, it has been compared to antihistamine drugs
- Those who suffer from Irritable Bowel Syndrome (IBS) sometimes experience intermittent constipation. MSM can sometimes help to reverse this problem.

The important thing to remember is that MSM, like many natural remedies, only takes effect after c
ontinued usage and often over a period of weeks.

Vitamin A

This vitamin is often included in nutritional programmes designed to help heal the lining of the gut. This is because vitamin A helps in the production of an antibody known as secretory IgA and a protective mucous. Both these substances act as a barrier against bacteria, parasites, yeast and food allergens, preventing them from making contact with the gut lining and being absorbed into the bloodstream where they can provoke immune responses.

Vitamin A also has a modulating role in preventing the release of too many inflammatory prostaglandins released in the presence of a food allergen. It is also very important for supporting the immune system, which it does by helping to maintain the health of the thymus gland (known as the immune system's master gland). Vitamin A is taken as a supplement at levels of up to 1,500mcg (micrograms) per day. **However, pregnant women and women who are likely to become pregnant must not take more than this as too much vitamin A may cause birth defects.** There is also a possibility of toxic effects if too much is taken. Signs of this can include dry, cracking skin (including cracking at the edge of the mouth), brittle nails, excessive hair loss, bleeding gums, weight loss, fatigue, irritability and nausea. Despite the dangers associated with vitamin A overdose, it is still a valuable component of a programme designed to alleviate the effects of food intolerance/allergy.

Vitamin C

Throughout the body, vitamin C is involved in many functions including the formation of collagen, which is so important for growth and repair of the cells that make up our tissues. It helps with allergies and intolerances on several levels, including the following:

- It neutralises many toxins, rendering them harmless. For example, as previously discussed, sodium nitrite (used as a colouring agent and preservative in some fish and meat products) can form carcinogenic compounds in the stomach called nitrosamines. Vitamin C is known to prevent their formation
- It helps to support the immune system
  The effect of numerous allergy- and intolerance-producing substances is reduced because it has a natural anti-histamine action
- To reduce the effects of histamine, some therapists recommend you take high levels of vitamin C as soon as you experience any ill effects from eating an offending food. This involves taking crystallised vitamin C at a dose of 1 teaspoon every hour until diarrhoea is produced. This indicates your vitamin C threshold has been reached. When this happens you need to cut back to ½ teaspoon every hour until you notice an improvement in your symptoms.

CAUTION!

If you have a history of kidney stones it's important that you take a magnesium supplement at a dose of 400mg per day while trying this method of vitamin C therapy. People with kidney disease should seek medical advice before taking Vitiman C, and pregnant women should avoid this approach.

Bromelain

This is an enzyme found in pineapples. It is often recommended as a supplement to help with protein digestion. It is frequently employed for its anti-inflammatory properties by nutritional therapists, though. In fact, it has been favourably compared to anti-inflammatory drugs such as aspirin and non-steroidal anti-inflammatories. Most research shows that the effect seems to be due to the action of bromelain on certain tissue hormones called eicosanoids. Some of these increase inflammation, while others decrease inflammation. Like anti-inflammatory drugs, bromelain appears to inhibit the pro-inflammatory hormones but unlike drugs, it has the advantage of being natural and free from potentially harmful side effects. Researchers investigating the anti-inflammatory effect of bromelain on eicosanoids, included Vellini, whose results, in a study that involved artificially induced inflammation in rats, seemingly indicate bromelain's effectiveness in reducing the inflammation.[1]

Used on its own, bromelain may help to minimise the effects of food intolerance when histamine is involved. Its effectiveness may be increased when used in conjunction with vitamin C and Omega 3 fatty acids.

CAUTION!

Because Bromelain acts a blood thinner, avoid it if you're taking anti-coagulant drugs.

1 Valleni, M, Desidera, D, Milanese, A, Orini, C, Daffonshio, L, Hernandez, A and Brunelli, G (1986) Arzheim-Forsch 36, 110

Aloe Vera

This is a cactus-like plant that is really a member of the lily family. It grows in countries with a warm climate and for centuries, it has been known by several cultures around the world as a powerful medicinal plant. Its succulent leaves are a source of aloe vera juice (the jelly-like substance present in the plant). The juice of the plant is consumed for its medicinal properties while the gel is often used topically for treating conditions such as sunburn.

As with the other supplements discussed in this chapter, Aloe vera has potent anti-inflammatory properties. Its healing and soothing effects have been observed when the juice or gel is applied to radiation and other types of burns and wounds. Similarly, the Aloe vera juice has been shown to be equally helpful when taken internally, this being due to its ability to reduce inflammation and heal the tissues that line the digestive tract.

The other major benefit of Aloe vera is its ability to increase the activity and effectiveness of the immune system. These two major properties make it a good addition to a programme designed to alleviate the effects of a food allergy or intolerance. What's more, the healing action on the epithelium cells that line the digestive tract may reduce a tendency to manifest food intolerances in the first place. One final advantage: the plant is known to possess anti-fungal properties and can be a good addition to an anti-Candida programme.

When selecting which aloe vera juice to take, it's important to select whole leaf extract, which has a more potent effect. The amount taken varies according to the level of treatment. In acute cases of food intolerance, I would suggest 50–100ml per day until symptoms diminish. After this a more moderate intake would comprise 25–50ml a day, taken between meals on an empty stomach.

Quercetin

This is a natural substance found in many fruits and vegetables. It has an anti-histamine effect and is therefore a valuable addition to the programme advocated here. Although naturally present in the type of foods recommended in this book, it is advisable for you to take a supplement in order to benefit from its effects. Most therapists recommend taking 500mg three times a day when suffering severe reactions and 500mg per day as a maintenance dose. It can be more effective combined with the other anti-inflammatory supplements or if this is too cost prohibitive, you can prioritise and take it with bromelain and vitamin C. For best results take 250–500mg of quercetin daily with at least 2 x 1000mg vitamin C tablets (preferably in a slow-release, low-acid form) and between 250–500mg of bromelain, three times daily.

Fruit and vegetables

When I was a teenager suffering from juvenile arthritis, fruits and vegetables proved to be my saviour. I discovered firsthand their potent anti-inflammatory effects. In fact, having completely revolutionised my diet so that the bulk of what I ate comprised of these foods, I not only experienced freedom from pain and swelling for the first time in months but I was also able to resume my sporting lifestyle and eventually qualified as a teacher of Physical Education. Mind you, this didn't come about without sacrifices because I did have to give up quite a few of my favourite foods including grains such as wheat.

Undoubtedly, fruit and vegetables can play a major role in helping to prevent food intolerances as well as alleviating their effects. This is not surprising because many contain significant supplies of quercetin, antioxidants and other useful plant compounds –one of the reasons why fruit and vegetables are mostly anti-inflammatory. Of course this is good news for allergy and food intolerance sufferers. Admittedly, if you are intolerant of any fruit and/or vegetables, you must omit them from your diet. Hopefully, though, there'll be plenty of others that you can use in their place.

Fruits and vegetables are also good anti-inflammatory foods because they form alkaline salts in the body. Sometimes people are confused: quite rightly, they observe that many fruits are acidic. This is true. However, although they enter the body as acids, fruits are then converted to alkaline salts. These salts have the amazing capacity to dislodge stored-up toxins in the body. Once dislodged from the tissues, toxins circulate in the blood before they are voided to the outside of the body through various channels of elimination – namely, the kidneys, faeces and the skin. That's why fruit and vegetables form the foundation of most detoxification programmes.

The problem that most people have is that they eat far too many acid-forming foods such as cheese, meats, most nuts, pulses and most grains. Enjoy too many of these foods and your system will become too acidic. But guess what? Acidity promotes inflammation and may well increase your allergic potential. The pH of blood is 7.4, which means that it's slightly alkaline. This is the reason why your diet should be based largely on the alkaline-forming fruit and vegetables, with the acid-forming foods eaten in lesser amounts. Therefore, the acid/alkaline balance should be:

65–70% alkaline-forming foods
30–35% acid-forming foods

Unfortunately, most of us get this the wrong way round and our bodies become too acidic. Below is a quick guide to the alkaline and acid-forming foods.

Acid-forming: Meat, fish, nuts (except almonds and coconut), most cheeses (except cottage cheese), most grains, plums, cranberries and olives.

Alkaline-forming: Most fruits and vegetables, including cabbage, cauliflower, broccoli, celery, lettuce, onions, root vegetables, tomatoes, apricots, apples, bananas, berries, figs, grapefruit, oranges, lemons, melon (all kinds), grapes, etc.

By basing your diet around alkaline-forming foods, you will reap the following benefits:

- Quicker recovery from the effects of food intolerance
- Reduced inflammation
- Lower toxic load due to the detoxifying effects of fruits and vegetables
- Stronger immune system
- Increased resistance to the development of intolerances
- Improved weight regulation

Healing the gut
Sometimes food intolerances and subsequent weight regulation problems can even be reversed if we focus on healing the lining of the gut. As already stated, a leaky gut can trigger off food allergies and intolerances. The good news is

that we can encourage the gut lining to heal itself as a result of using the following supplements:

Digestive enzymes: Some sufferers report an improvement in their symptoms when they begin taking digestive enzymes with their meals. These enzymes help to support the enzymes already produced in your digestive system. As their name suggests, they digest foods, breaking them down into simpler substances that your body can use for growth, repair and maintenance – for example, proteins into amino acids. The key enzymes are: lipase for fat digestion, amylase for the digestion of starches and protease for protein digestion. Sometimes, when taken with meals, these additional enzymes help to ensure that foods are more completely digested. This reduces the chances of partly digested food particles triggering off immune reactions. In other words, digestive enzymes may help reduce the occurrence of food intolerances. There are implications concerning weight loss too because more complete digestion of foods may reduce the likelihood of food being stored as fats.

Digestive enzymes can be taken as tablets or capsules. Some are derived entirely from plants and are therefore suitable for vegetarians and vegans. Others, such as pancreatin, are derived from animals.

CAUTION!
Do not take digestive enzymes if pregnant or breast-feeding

Caprylic acid: This is a short-chain fatty acid found in breast milk and coconuts. It is known to help heal the gut and promote the growth of healthy bacteria. For this reason, it's a supplement that is often included in an anti-Candida programme. Because of its gut-healing properties it may help to prevent or alleviate food intolerances.

Glutamine: This important amino acid is synthesised in the body; however it is known to be excellent in supporting the immune system as well as being a primary source of fuel for the cells lining the small intestine. In helping these cells to proliferate, glutamine is known to help heal a leaky gut. These properties obviously make it a valuable supplement in terms of treatment for alleviating and even eradicating food intolerances.

Glutamine can be taken as powder mixed with water. The recommended dose is around 12g daily, with 6g being taken in the morning and 6g last thing at night, preferably on an empty stomach.

Probiotics: As discussed earlier in this book, probiotics (or healthy bacteria) can be extremely beneficial to the health of your digestive system. Apart from helping to keep pathogenic organisms such as yeasts in check, they help reduce your allergic potential by supporting the immune system in addition to many other useful functions.

The best way to take them is in the form of capsules or powder. The latter is mixed with water and taken on an empty stomach. Most manufacturers such as Biocare recommend you take one capsule twice daily with food and most formulae consist of a combination of acidophilus and bifido bifidum bacteria, with a billion or more of each strain of bacteria. Don't take them with hot liquids – this will kill the bacteria.

Prebiotics: These are naturally occurring substances that help to feed the healthy bacteria in the digestive tract. A good example is FOS (fructo-oligo-saccherides), a special kind of carbohydrate derived from some vegetables which encourages the growth of 'friendly' bacteria. This is termed a prebiotic effect. Because of this, it's often recommended as an important component of an anti-Candida and gut-healing programme. Prebiotics are often added to probiotics to enhance their action.

FOS usually comes in powdered form and the recommended dosage for adults is 5g initially, followed by 10g daily as a maintenance dose. It can cause initial bloating and loose stools but this usually settles down with continued use. If bloating persists, discontinue and consult your doctor.

18

The Big Fat Mystery solved

Having read the previous chapters, you'll now be aware that food intolerances can be closely linked to poor metabolism, water retention and weight gain. Nevertheless, by addressing other key areas such as the importance of healthy eating and minimising the level of toxins in your body, you'll also understand that food intolerance and weight gain form just part of a whole range of inter-related influences on the body and mind, all of which can wield an enormous impact on your ability to achieve good health and long-term freedom from weight gain. I use the term 'inter-related' because all the factors that have been addressed so far can impact on one another and that's why I have endeavoured to stress the importance of a truly holistic approach towards food intolerances and possible weight issues. The following plan of action brings together all of the key elements within this book. It is, if you like, your prescription for weight loss and wellbeing:

Your action plan

- Identify your food intolerances
- Eliminate any offending foods from your diet
- Rotate foods to which you are less sensitive.

Diet:

- Try to eat plenty of fruit and vegetables, 50% of which should be in their raw state
- Eat at least one large salad per day and include a wide variety of ingredients
- Include the whole grains that you can tolerate
- Eat oily fish (not breaded or smoked) 2–3 times weekly
- If you eat poultry and meat, opt for chicken and occasionally lamb and lamb's liver. Choose organic whenever possible
- Eat raw nuts and seeds (not roasted or salted) in moderation. Pumpkin, hemp and flaxseeds are very beneficial. Ground flaxseeds are the best plant source of Omega 3 fats
- Reduce or eliminate your consumption of dairy products
- Try to drink freshly extracted fruit and vegetable juices
- If possible, include freshly sprouted nuts, seeds, vegetables and grains in your diet.

Exercise

Aim to engage in some form of exercise at least three times each week. This can take many forms, including team sports, swimming, yoga, cycling, working out in a gym or even just walking briskly.

Pollution

- Try to minimise your exposure to exhaust fumes (for example, walk along less polluted routes wherever possible)

- Avoid using aluminium cookware
- Eliminate or restrict your intake of artificial additives
- Use filtered or pure bottled water (the latter from low-land sources wherever possible) for drinking and cooking
- Follow the dietary advice above and eat organic foods wherever possible
- Use cosmetics and cleaning materials that contain only natural ingredients whenever possible.

Your supplement prescription for healing the gut

* = Avoid if pregnant or lactating

- Digestive enzymes: derived from animal or plant sources*
- Dosage: One capsule with each meal
- Caprylic acid: Usually comes in the form of capsules or tablets*
- Dosage: 300mg twice daily with meals
- Glutamine: 12g daily divided into two 6g doses dissolved in water, one to be taken last thing at night and the other first thing in the morning*
- Probiotics: Choose a formula containing at least 1 billion viable organisms per capsule, with an equal amount of acidophilus and bifidum (see Useful Information, page 303 for the best sources of this)
- Dosage: One capsule twice daily with food
- Prebiotics: Fructo-oligo-saccherides (FOS) is the most commonly used. Available as a powder
- Dosage: 10g per day as a maintenance dose
- Aloe Vera: Best taken as aloe vera juice but opt for whole leaf extract*
- Dosage: 50ml per day on an empty stomach.

Nutrients for everyday maintenance and support

High strength multivitamin and mineral formula: This is a good source of the key vitamins and minerals needed to support your immune system, protect against pollutants and provide the nutrients required for digestive function.

CAUTION

women who have not yet reached the menopause should check the level of vitamin A in a multivitamin formula to ensure that it doesn't exceed the recommended dose of 1,500mcg (note: mcg indicates micrograms, not grams)

- Dosage: Usually one tablet per day taken with food
- Vitamin C: A great all-rounder. Helps support the immune system and acts as an anti-toxin
- Dosage: One slow-release 1,000mg tablet taken in the morning and one at night. If pregnant, limit this to one 1,000mg daily.
- Cold-pressed flaxseed oil: Good for weight loss as it speeds up the metabolism. Most people are deficient in Omega 3 fats but have too much of Omega 6, which is why I suggest taking flaxseed oil for the first six months to redress the balance between Omega 3 and Omega 6 fats. This is followed by a formula that will provide you with a good balance between Omega 3 and 6 essential fats
- Dosage: Three tablespoons daily with meals for the first six months followed by a balanced oil blend such as Udo's Choice or Higher Nature's Essential Balance.

Anti-inflammatory prescription

These supplements can be taken for one to two months as a short-term solution to counteract inflammation produced from food intolerance. * = Avoid if pregnant or lactating

- MSM: Usually available in tablet form*
- Dosage: One 500mg tablet twice daily with food
- Bromelain: Comes in tablet or capsule form*
- Dosage: One 500mg tablet or the equivalent in capsules twice daily between meals
- Quercitin: Usually available in tablets or capsules*
- Dosage: One 500mg tablet or the equivalent in capsules twice daily between meals

A word about supplementation

I am aware that the comprehensive supplement programme described above may be cost-prohibitive for some readers. Therefore, should you wish to limit your intake to just a few supplements, I recommend you treat the high-strength multivitamin and mineral formula (see Useful Information for best sources, page 303), vitamin C and the probiotics as priorities. If your diet consists of an abundance of fresh fruits, raw vegetables and juices (preferably organic, whenever possible), this will provide many of the nutrients required on a daily basis.

CAUTION!

If you have a medical condition or are pregnant or breast feeding, consult your doctor before taking supplements. Because Bromelain acts as a blood thinner, it should be avoided by those taking anti-coagulant drugs.

Conclusion

Hopefully, if you have embraced the principles in this book, you will now be aware that you have an invaluable opportunity at your disposal. In fact, you have been equipped with all the tools necessary to enhance your ability to tackle allergies and intolerances, gain more energy, enjoy improved hea;th and create the conditions in which you are in control of your weight.

Of course, it's one thing being given the tools, and quite another to use them effectively. Give it a try! The rewards associated with your health and wellbeing are truly priceless. Good luck!

Appendix I
Index of recipes

Appendix II
Food family classifications

The chances are that if you react to one member of a food family there is an increased risk that you will react to other members of the same family in the same way unless you have been tested for those foods and have shown no reaction. For example, if you react to kidney beans, you may also react to other members of the legume family such as lentil, liquorice, pea, peanut, senna, soya, tapioca and carob. The following list of classifications will help you when planning your rotation diet.

Family name	Foods in the family
PLANTS	
Banana	Arrowroot, banana, ginger, plantain, turmeric, vanilla
Beech	Beechnut, chestnut
Beet	Beet, chard, spinach, sugar beet
Berry	Blackberry, boysenberry, loganberry, raspberry, strawberry
Birch	Hazelnut, wintergreen
Buckwheat	Buckwheat, rhubarb, sorrel
Carrot	Angelica, caraway, carrot, celery, chervil, coriander, cumin, dill, fennel, parsley, parsnip
Cashew	Cashew, mango, pistachio
Citrus	Citron, grapefruit, lemon, lime, mandarin, orange, tangerine
Composites	Artichoke, chamomile, chicory, dandelion, endive, lettuce, safflower, salsify, sunflower, tarragon
Fungi	Mushroom, truffle, yeast
Gourd	Courgette, cucumber, gherkin, melon (honeydew), pumpkin, squash, watermelon
Grape	Cream of tartar, grape, raisin, sultana
Grass	Bamboo shoots, barley, corn, millet, oat, rice, rye, sugar cane, sorghum, wheat
Heather	Blueberry
Laurel	Avocado, bay leaf, cinnamon, sassafras
Legume	Bean, carob, lentil, liquorice, pea, peanut, senna, soya, tapioca
Lily	Asparagus, chive, garlic, leek, onion, shallot
Madder	Coffee
Mint	Basil, bergamot, lavender, lemon balm, marjoram, mint, oregano, rosemary, sage, thyme
Mulberry	Breadfruit, fig, hop, mulberry
Mustard	Broccoli, Brussels sprouts, cabbage, cauliflower, Chinese leaves, cress, horseradish, kale, kohlrabi, mustard radish, rapeseed, turnip, watercress
Olive	Olive
Palm	Coconut, date, palm, sago

Pineapple	Pineapple
Potato (Nightshades)	Aubergine, cayenne pepper, chilli pepper, paprika, pepper, potato, sesame, tahini, tobacco, tomato
Rose	Apple, cider, crab-apple, pear, rosehip
Rosestone family	Almond, apricot, cherry, nectarine, peach plum, prune, quince, sloe
Saxifrage	Blackcurrant, currant, gooseberry
Stericula	Chocolate, cocoa, cola
Tea	Tea
Verbena	Lemon verbena
Walnut	Butternut, pecan nut, walnut

FOWL

Dove	Pigeon
Duck	Duck, goose
Grouse	Grouse, partridge
Guinea fowl	Guinea fowl
Pheasant	Chicken, chicken egg, peafowl, pheasant, quail
Turkey	Turkey

MAMMALS

Bovid	Beef, buffalo, cow, cow cheese, cream, feta, gelatine, goat, goat cheese, goat milk, lamb, milk, Roquefort, sheep, sheep cheese, veal, whey, yoghurt
Deer	Caribou, elk moose, reindeer, venison
Hare	Hare, rabbit
Swine	Pork

Seafood:	
Crustacean	Crab, crayfish, lobster, prawn, shrimp
Mollusc	Abalone, clam, cockle, mussel, oyster, scallop, snail, squid
Octopus	Octopus

FRESHWATER FISH

Bass	Bass, perch (white), yellow bass
Herring	Shad
Minnow	Carp, chub

Perch	Perch (yellow), red snapper
Pike	Pickerel, pike
Salmon	Salmon, trout
Smelt	Smelt
Sturgeon	Caviar, sturgeon
Sunfish	Black bass

SALTWATER FISH

Anchovy	Anchovy
Codfish	Cod, cod liver oil, haddock, hake, pollock
Eel	Eel
Flounder	Flounder, halibut, plaice, sole, turbot
Mackerel	Bonito, mackerel, tuna
Mullet	Mullet
Porgy	Bream, porgy
Salmon	Sea trout
Scorpionfish	Ocean perch, rockfish
Sea bass	Grouper, sea bass
Sea catfish	Catfish
Sea herring	Herring, pilchard, sardine
Skate	Skate
Honey	Natural honey contains multiple plant pollens. Commercial honey frequently contains sugar

Thanks to Yorktest.com for their kind permission to reproduce this food table.

Appendix III
Useful information

Food intolerance testing

Signs of Life electro-dermal testing provide services to help detect food intolerances, environmental sensitivities such as house-dust mite, printer's ink, etc., heavy metals, vitamin and mineral deficiencies, digestive function, parasites and hormone levels.

For bookings call Signs of Life on 01732 508527 or 0778 8710 667. Or email bio_cure@hotmail.com. For further information, visit www.fooddetective.co.uk.

For further information on this type of testing, look at the Biomeridian website: www.biomeridian.com and www.vitalitydirect.net.

YorkTest laboratories test for food intolerances. They sell a home testing kit for food and chemical intolerances. Contact them to order a home test kit on freephone: 0800 074 6185 or via their website: www.yorktest.com. View their website on: www.yorktest.com.

Test for Intestinal Permeability (leaky gut)

Contact Individual Well-being Diagnostic Laboratories: call +44 (0)20 8336 7750 or visit their website: www.iwdl.net.

Eating disorders

If you think you may be suffering from an eating disorder, contact The Eating Disorders Association, 1st Floor, Wensum House, 103 Prince of Wales Road, Norwich NR1 1DW. Adult helpline: 0845 634 1414; youthline: 0845 634 765.

Recommended reading

Cairney, E., *The Sprouters Handbook*, Argyll Publishing, reprinted 2002.

de Vries, J., *The Jan de Vries Guide to Health and Vitality*, Trafalgar Square, 2006.

Ersamus, Dr. U., *Fats That Heal Fats That Kill*, Alive Books, 1987/1994.

Francis, R., with Cotton, K., *Never Be Sick Again*, Health Communications, Inc., 2002.

Graham, Dr. Douglas N., *On Nutrition and Physical Performance: A Handbook for Athletes and Fitness Enthusiasts* (www.foodnsport.com).

Graham, Dr. Douglas., *Grain Damage*, Food N Sport, 2005

Holford P., *New Optimum Nutrition Bible*, Piatkus Books, 2004.

Jacobs, G., *Beat Candida Through Diet*, Vermillion, 1997.

Oski, A. Frank, *Don't Drink Your Milk*, Teach Services, 1992.

Statham, B., *The Chemical Maze Shopping Companion*, Summersdale Publishers Ltd., 2006.

Vale, J., *The Juicemaster's Ultimate Fast Food: Discover the Power of Raw Juice*, HarperCollins, 2003.

Recommended supplement companies
Herbal remedies:
Bioforce (UK) Ltd: 01294 277344 or email:
enquiries@bioforce.co.uk.

Health supplements:
Biocare: For sales, telephone: 0121 4333727 Email:
sales@biocare.co.uk website: www.BioCare.co.uk.
Higher Nature: 01435 884668 or email: info@higher-
nature.co.uk.
Solgar: For your nearest supplier, telephone Solgar on 01442
890355. Website: www.solgar.com.

Recommended natural cosmetics
Dr. Hauschka Skin Care: For enquiries contact:
enquiries@drhauschka.co.uk. Telephone: 01386 791022.
Environ Products: Call Health products For Life on +44
(0)20 8874 8038, website: www.healthproductsforlife.com.
For international enquiries, ring +2721 683 1034 or visit
environ@iafrica.com.
Green People (organic skincare). Visit:
www.greenpeople.co.uk or email:
sales@theremustbeabetterway.co.uk.
Higher Nature: (see Health Supplements, above).
Weleda Skin Care Products: www.weleda.com.

Useful organisations
Allergy UK: A charity that supports people who suffer from
allergies or chemical sensitivities. Their website is a good
source of information on allergies and specialised products
for allergy sufferers. Visit: www.allergyuk.org or call their
helpline on: +44 (0)1322 619864.

The British Association of Nutritional Therapists (BANT):
For a list of registered practitioners in your area, email
administrator@bant.org.uk or telephone: 08706 0611284.
The British Naturopathic Association: For a list of reputable
naturopaths in your locality, telephone: 0870 745 6984.

If you live outside the UK then seek advice from a
recognized national organisation.

Information on food safety is provided by the European
Union and European Commission:
http://europa.eu/pol/food/index_en.htm;
www.eurunion.org/policyareas/food.htm.
The American Dietetic Association provides nutritional
information and a registry of dieticians throughout the
USA. www.eatright.org
Information on all aspects of pesticide use is available from
the Pesticides Residue Committee:
www.pesticides.gov.uk/prc_home.asp
A comprehensive eco-aware site is www.mindfully.org,
which includes information on health, particularly on the
subject of pesticides and other potentially harmful
substances. Though based in the UK, their scope is global
and links to articles in English are listed.
The Australian Department of Health and Ageing provides
statistical information on health research as well as links to
health resources in Australia and worldwide.
www.health.gov.au.
The Institute of Optimum Nutritoin (ION) offers a three-
year degree course in nutritional therapy. There is a clinic, a
list of practitioners across the UK and overseas an
information service and a quarterly journal. www.ion.ac.uk